STOP THE NIGHTMARES OF TRAUMA

Thought Field Therapy (TFT)
The Power Therapy for the 21st Century

Roger J. Callahan, Ph.D.

and

Joanne Callahan, MBA (Health Care)

ISBN Number 1-57087-505-7

Library of Congress Catalog Card Number 99-76342

Professional Press
Chapel Hill, NC 27515-4371

Manufactured in the United States of America
00 01 02 03 04   10 9 8 7 6 5 4 3 2 1

DEDICATION

We dedicate this work to our grandchildren
Jennifer, Ryan, Caitlin, Haley, Tessa, Charlie and Will

RJC and JC

DISCLAIMER

All material presented herein is provided for educational purposes only and may not be construed as medical or psychological advice or instruction. No action or inaction should be taken based solely on the contents herein; instead, readers or viewers should consult appropriate health professionals on any matter relating to their health. This information and the opinions provided here are believed to be accurate and sound, based on the best judgment available to the authors. Readers or viewers who fail to consult with appropriate health authorities assume the risk of any injuries.

ACKNOWLEDGEMENTS

It is easy to confuse Thought Field Therapy (TFT) with acupuncture or Applied Kinesiology. Actually it is neither, but without the preceding work and discoveries in these fields my (RJC's) discoveries never would have been possible (see the Chapter Notes on Discovery). Therefore, I wish to express my profound appreciation to the unknown genius in the Orient who first discovered the energy meridians that travel throughout the human body. Also, I want to acknowledge my great appreciation to George Goodheart, DC, the genius who discovered and developed Applied Kinesiology (AK), for without his discoveries, mine would not have been possible.

I also wish to thank David Walther, DC, and Robert Blaich, DC, for teaching me AK and in welcoming this psychologist to their hundred-hour course in that subject many years ago. Their grasp and appreciation of my discovery of psychological reversal (discovered *before* I took the course) was encouraging at a time when I was not receiving much encouragement. Thought Field Therapy, however is not AK. The AK principals and I would agree on this.

I have never received outside financial support for my years of research and development of TFT. All my work has been made possible by my clients who had faith in, or at least were willing to try a method which seemed quite strange but nevertheless yielded powerful results—I thank them for putting up with the seeming strangeness of the procedures.

Our trainees, and especially those trained in Voice Technology™ (VT), have been a delight to work with and we are grateful for their support. I would like to acknowledge especially Dr. Stephen Daniel, VT; Dr. Gale Joslin, VT; Liz Joslin, VT; Yoshinori Takasaki, MD, VT; Dr. Caroline Sakai, VT; Monica Pignotti, VT; Dr. Jill Strunk, VT; Dr. Norma Shenck, VT; Dr. Mark Steinberg, VT; Dr. Jennifer Edwards; Dr. Luis Jorge Gonzalez; and Richard Petty, MD.

We would like to thank Ryan Tannascoli for his illustrations.

We have received editorial help for this project and we would especially like to thank Dr. Jill Strunk, VT; Monica Pignotti, VT; Dr. Mark Steinberg, Curtis Morris, and Ginny Turner for their special help and attention, as well as editorial suggestions. Remaining errors are the sole responsibility of the authors.

RJC and JC
LaQuinta, California, 1999

CONTENTS

FOREWORD

Much of human suffering in the world today is due to traumatic events. Man-made events such as war and crime, as well as natural disasters from earthquakes to hurricanes all leave their victims in pain, tortured with vivid past memories and recurring nightmares.

My years of teaching seminars to accelerate personal and professional development and enhance self-esteem have shown me how fragile we human beings are and how deeply affected we are by our fears and past traumas. As a result, many of the stories in our Chicken Soup for the Soul® Series are centered around the courage needed to overcome or respond to some sort of trauma in our lives.

I have used Dr. Callahan's simple techniques for overcoming fears and phobias, the Five Minute Phobia Cure, in my teaching and seminars for nearly ten years. Often, eliminating a simple fear such as fear of public speaking can go a long way to improving an individual's self-esteem and increasing the expression of their innate potential.

Unfortunately, up until now, there has never really been a brief and effective self-help procedure for past traumas. Healing from traumas usually takes time. Suffering often continues for many, many years as the victim relives the event over and over again. Children often suffer the most.

In this new book, Dr. Callahan offers a completely new theory as to why we have recurrent nightmares and why we suffer for extended periods following most traumatic events. He tells us that most of this suffering is needless and gives us step-by-step procedures to alleviate the pain, nightmares, and stress that haunt us.

Stop the Nightmares of Trauma, for the first time in history, gives us a simple, painless way to reduce and even eliminate the painful emotions and nightmares from our past traumas. We now have at our fingertips a safe and natural technique to help reduce the suffering of trauma victims throughout the world.

Jack Canfield
President, Self-Esteem Seminars and
Co-Author, Chicken Soup for the Soul® Series

NOTE

When the words "I," "me" or "my" are used they refers to the primary author, RJC.

The descriptive term (name) Thought Field Therapy (TFT) cannot be trademarked. Therefore, in order to distinguish the authentic and standardized TFT from the numerous diluted copies, we sometimes use the term Callahan Techniques® TFT or CTTFT. Callahan Techniques® was the original name during the first fifteen years of development of the procedures now referred to as Thought Field Therapy. Therefore, Callahan Techniques® (CT) identifies the originator or source.

After careful thought during its development, I came up with the name TFT. But now, the term by itself has lost its significance since individuals who do not clearly understand this work are applying the name TFT to much-diluted, hybridized and less-effective versions.

CHAPTER 1

HOW TFT VIEWS TRAUMA

I maintain that most of the treatments used to help trauma victims today, which entail suffering and reliving the emotional experience, are harmful and trauma-inducing in their own right. It makes no difference that numerous so-called experts acclaim these outmoded procedures—they fail the scientific test; they are experiments that not only do not work, but in fact cause harm. Generations of suffering people have been wrongly taught that suffering is necessary and that they must endure a process of suffering.

Those who do not wish to endure emotional suffering now have a choice. My value is that it is desirable to reduce or eliminate suffering as much as possible. Some professionals have criticized my work because they believe it is important for people to suffer. I do not agree.

When anesthesia was first discovered there was an uproar among some factions (men) who objected to women not having pain in childbirth. They cited the Bible

1

ble pre-dated the dis-
 at Eastern Michigan
 David Palmer (Speech
 an operation first be-
 re were objections from
 araphrased a part of the
 put asunder, let no man

s that the individual should have a choice, if poss... We now offer a choice. It is now possible to put Humpty Dumpty together again and end the trauma.

In this book you will learn how to repeat some of the experiments based upon my discoveries relating to psychological trauma. Professionals have already successfully repeated this experiment on trauma many thousands of times all over the world. Now you will be able to repeat the experiment in the style of Mr. Wizard, who teaches principles of science on television. Although Mr. Wizard is geared for children it is one of my favorite television shows.

You will learn in this book how to eliminate the nightmares associated with traumas and also the painful psychological aftereffects of terrible and upsetting experiences. If you can't wait, you can go right to the chapter called How to Eliminate the Nightmares and Pain of Trauma and begin to practice the procedures. However, it is important to read all the material in the book in order to gain an understanding of TFT and to be able to do a better job of helping others.

Trauma refers to having a terrible experience. A phobia is an unwarranted fear. Trauma is different from a phobia. The upset in trauma is a normal upset in response to a terrible situation. A phobic person can have a traumatic experience due to his particular and unique, however unwarranted, fear. Most others do not share this unrealistic fear and hence would not be traumatized by the same fear event. However, everyone will be quite upset by a trauma.

Traumas are commonly due to loss or negative event, e.g., losing a loved one, rape, mugging, robbery, accidents, war, industrial accidents, abuse, losing your job, school bombings, acts of terrorism, death of a loved one, getting a severe illness, and other bad events. Even witnessing or hearing about such events can have traumatic consequences, especially if the trauma happens to someone you know and care about.

Post-traumatic stress refers to stress that is delayed, perhaps for years. However, there is no difference in the way we view or treat trauma based on the time factor. Trauma is treated in the same way in TFT whether or not it is a problem right after the event or whether time passes prior to the upset. I once treated a concentration camp victim a half a century after the experience. However, his stress had been constant and not delayed.

Most psychological problems such as phobias are bewildering to people who have them. The central characteristic of a phobia is that it is an unrealistic fear. The person *knows* it is an absurd fear but nevertheless cannot help being afraid. If anything, this knowledge merely adds humiliation to the fear. Obsessions, addictions, distortions of reality—all are types of problems considered abnormal.

It makes more sense that an abnormal fear, say of bugs, should be curable rather than the severe upset over a terrible situation. Trauma is a unique class of problems, for it consists of a perfectly normal, appropriate, emotionally disturbed reaction to an objectively terrible situation or event. There are people who overreact to trauma but they also overreact to a normally upsetting situation.

I find it especially interesting and intriguing that it is possible to banish all traces of emotional upset over a very real objective trauma. Until I made this discovery I thought that only time would partially heal traumas, sometimes taking many years of prolonged suffering.

Recently I treated a woman whose boyfriend had committed suicide. She was naturally very upset, unable to function very well and was constantly in severe psychological pain. Immediately after the treatment she felt strong in the face of this tragedy and was again able to function and carry out her job. The ease and power of this simple treatment suggests that we have a healing power within us that only awaits a simple correct procedure in order for the healing data to kick in and take us into a higher state of health. Psychologists Carl Rogers and Abraham Maslow suggested many years ago that we all have this power within us, and TFT supports their views by making this power clearly evident to any interested observer. If Rogers and Maslow were alive, I am confident they would be shocked and pleased to see this power released with such ease and regularity through Thought Field Therapy (TFT).

I interpret my therapy results, which you will be able to reproduce, as evidence that Nature gives us a license to be relatively free of intense emotional upset from very real, objectively horrible events; otherwise it would not be so easy.

REMOVING THE EMOTIONAL EFFECTS OF TRAUMA DOES NOT CHANGE REALITY

TFT can now easily remove the emotional effects of trauma, but the reality of a trauma, alas, remains. However, this reality can now be completely stripped of disruptive and disturbing emotional effects. Though important, effective therapy cannot change reality. If, for example, parents lose a child, this reality must be lived with for the rest of their lives. There is no way to change the grim reality, and until recently there was no way to change the emotional hurt and pain. The loss will remain real, but one may become strong in the face of a grim reality.

Recently an acquaintance informed me of the recent loss of a much-loved 19-year-old nephew to suicide. The suicide was a response to love loss—his girlfriend had just broken up with him. Love pain is one of the most disruptive of emotions. Murder and suicides are not rare in this turbulent emotion. I helped the acquaintance who was suffering terribly from the grief of loss. It took only three minutes to accomplish this result. The extreme look of pain on her face was immediately gone. Of course, the loss is permanent but the severe emotional pain is completely gone. Perhaps, if the nephew had been aware of this simple treatment, it's quite possible his life could have been saved. This powerful trauma algorithm is so easy to do that everyone should know it for a psychological first aid procedure.

It is a common observation that severely handicapped people ought to be depressed over their situation but most, fortunately, are not. Depression and other emotions, as viewed by TFT, are not exclusively the result of a reality condition but rather the result of what we call perturbations in a thought field. When viewed this way we can understand how it is possible to treat severe traumas, not by changing reality, but rather by eliminating the fundamental cause of the suffering.

THE EASE OF THE TRAUMA TREATMENT DOES NOT ELIMINATE THE IMPORTANT CONCEPT OF JUSTICE

That we can treat traumas with relative ease should not obscure the fact that victims are entitled to justice. One professional expressed concern to me that if no one was upset over a rape, then rape might become acceptable. Emotional upset should not be the relevant standard but rather the criminality of the act. We can, and should, pursue justice without remaining unnecessarily upset. There is an old saying attributed to the Kennedys: "Don't get mad, get even." We can all be outraged over rape or other such crimes and pursue justice diligently without becoming personally devastated over the matter; in fact, we probably will do a better job of carrying out justice, the stronger and more resolute we can remain.

CHAPTER 2

DISCOVERY OF THE TRAUMA TREATMENT

I believe the development of new treatments to relieve PTSD (Post-Traumatic Stress Disorder) is of the highest priority.

Martin Seligman, Ph.D.
Former President, American Psychological Association

I n Shakespeare's *Macbeth*, the question is asked: "Canst thou not pluck from the mind a rooted sorrow?" In the scene where this question is asked, Macbeth is talking with Lady Macbeth's doctor and asks if knowledge is available to help Lady Macbeth get over the trauma about which she is obsessing. The only answer to this question until recent years was no. Before the development of TFT, psychological science had no effective way to "pluck from the mind a rooted sorrow." You can directly experience this therapy phenomenon by experimenting with TFT using the treatment provided in this book. In doing so, you will find that there is now a surprisingly effective way to pluck the disturbing emotions associated with sorrow from the mind.

My first development in TFT was a rapid, easily replicable cure for most phobias (Callahan, 1981, 1996). It was an astonishing finding, because I first started attempting to treat phobias in 1950. About 30 years later I discovered this remarkable cure for phobias. Although I had been practicing psychotherapy since 1950 and had heard and read about phobias being cured, I had never actually seen it done. Since I found it relatively easy to cure a phobia (Callahan, 1985), I wondered if I could eliminate fears and distress based upon a traumatic experience.

Hopeless Cancer

A client came to me because she was in a constant state of near panic, fear, hurt, terror, and psychological pain. Her doctor had told her she had less than a year to live due to a severe and rapidly growing cancer. Two other physicians confirmed the diagnosis. She and her husband flew to California for still another expert opinion. The physician in California confirmed the bad news and suggested she try the new psychotherapy treatment I had been developing to alleviate her upset over this terrible reality. Her upset, in the face of this terrible reality, seemed perfectly normal to me. This was quite a different situation from most people who came to me for help. Her fear and upset were based on a realistically terrible condition. The challenge was, would I be able to find a treatment to help this unfortunate person?

When she came to see me, she was hysterical and sobbing profusely. There was no need to ask her to think about the problem as we usually do—she was obsessed with the cruel reality. I tried the treatment and the severe emotional distress and fear completely vanished in mere moments! She was crying and sobbing the whole time in my office until after the treatment. Nevertheless, during the treatment I asked her to think about the terrible verdict given to check the effectiveness of the treatment and make sure I did not merely momentarily distract her (an idea that now seems ludicrous). During the treatment I repeated to her what her doctors told her. After the treatment was finished I asked how she felt. "Well," she said, "I certainly don't like it, but my upset and fear seem to be gone. I feel surprisingly strong in the face of this terrible thing."

TWO PARTICULARLY HORRIBLE RAPES

Any rape is a terrible and traumatic experience. Usually, the victims' horror continues long after the rape, and is sometimes aggravated by legal and other procedures to which the rape victim may be subject. Soon after the cancer case I had the opportunity to work with two women who had experienced not just the usual terrible rape but particularly horrible rapes.

Gang Prisoner. An attractive client informed me that she was unable to date since her rape ten years earlier. She told a frightening story of the horrible event. She was recently divorced and had a four-year-old child. Four gang members had broken into her apartment and held her prisoner for a week while they took turns raping her. She said the worst part was they continually threatened to kill her extremely frightened child. Nightmares of this terrible incident continued to plague her. The rape haunted her continually and she was almost constantly upset. Although she wished she could be free to date, she couldn't due to the severe and constant distress of this past trauma.

Here was another example of an objectively terrible situation where disturbing emotions appeared to be a perfectly normal response to a monstrously horrible situation. Nevertheless, within a minute of the treatment, all traces of her upset vanished. Follow-up over four years revealed there was no return of the upset and no recurrence of nightmares.

A Creep in the Attic. Helen traveled some distance to see if relief might be possible for her continuing problem which had been unresponsive to ordinary psychotherapy. Her chiropractor had heard of the work I was doing and suggested that she try to see if I could help rid her of her constant suffering. Her story sounded like a horror movie. She was very happily married with two young children and very much in love with her husband. Her husband was on extended overseas military duty on a navy ship, and she did not want to burden him with the following horror story.

A man broke into her house and raped her. She reported this to the police and the man was arrested. However, he was out on bail soon after the arrest. A few nights later, she heard noises in her attic and she called the police. She saw the man who raped her escape. The police did not capture him. He was still free when she came to see me. Obviously she was an emotional wreck and did not know what to do. I urged her to contact her husband and get the ball rolling to get him home as soon as possible. I assured her that both he and the military would understand the necessity of this. In the meantime, the trauma treatment eliminated her emotional distress over the terrible events. She obviously did not forget these events nor did she repress the absolute horror of these events, but after treatment she was strong in the face of this grim reality.

Since I could eliminate most phobias with ease and now I could eliminate the negative effects of trauma, it seemed I had discovered the coding system or healing data for negative emotions, whether they were rational and appropriate (traumas) or irrational and inappropriate (phobias).

CHAPTER 3

HOW TO STOP THE NIGHTMARES AND PAIN OF TRAUMA: THE TFT ALGORITHM (RECIPE) FOR TRAUMA

Science is the belief in the ignorance of experts.

Richard Feynman
Nobel Laureate in Physics

I n a celebrated lecture to physics undergraduates at Cornell University, Professor Richard Feynman elaborated on the quote above. He said, "If it [a new scientific law] disagrees with experiment, it's wrong! In that simple statement is the key to science. It doesn't make any difference how beautiful your guess is, it doesn't make any difference how smart you are, who made the guess or what his name is, if it disagrees with experiment it's wrong; that's all there is to it."

IMPORTANT!!! Please keep in mind that the treatment presented here is for trauma and not for other problems such as phobias, which are an irrational fear.[1] The treatment for phobias is similar and is presented after the trauma treatment below.

INCIDENT

On the first day of one of my diagnostic trainings I asked the assembled group how many had tried TFT before coming to the training. Most hands went up. I asked if anyone there had been unsuccessful. It is unheard of to hear of no success with this powerful procedure. A high level professional person who had traveled from across the world to attend my training said that he had been unsuccessful with my trauma treatment. I was quite surprised by this report and asked him to join me at lunch. I asked him to please tell me exactly what he was doing to treat trauma and much to my surprise he described to me, my phobia algorithm. I said, "No wonder you had trouble, that is not the correct procedure for trauma!"

All of the TFT algorithms have been found through what I call *causal diagnosis.* Over two decades of treating thousands of patients with causal diagnosis, common pat-

---

[1] For those interested, we offer a TFT Causal Diagnostic Home Study Course (see back of book, it contains all TFT algorithms for many problems including phobias, depression, anxiety, and most other problems, even jet lag). The person who masters TFT Causal Diagnosis is able to find the precise treatment needed and will most often find algorithms unnecessary.

terns or algorithms have emerged. These have now been tested on many people, both in self-help applications and with thousands of trained professionals throughout the world.

My first trauma victim was cured, believe it or not, by doing nothing more than tapping the beginning of the eyebrow. However, upon trying this same simple procedure on others with traumas, I quickly found that most were not helped this easily. I had to make further discoveries to increase the success rate. Each discovery was tested for efficacy on my trauma clients; this allowed me to quickly develop further treatments and allow me to help more people.

The algorithm for trauma presented below has been tested on thousands of people and the success rate is quite good—about 80% of traumatized people are helped with this recipe or algorithm.

I have discovered and developed a number of different TFT treatments, called algorithms, for different problems. A TFT algorithm is a recipe or treatment formula for a particular problem that has been found to be effective for a high percentage of people. It is through my unique causal diagnostic procedures that we can find exactly what treatment an individual needs. I tested each aspect or section of the treatment on many people before I declared it to be generally successful. The trauma algorithm has now been tested all over the world.

We urge you to study the trauma treatment and begin by applying it to yourself. We all have past traumas of varying intensity, such as being rejected, especially in a love relationship, failing a class, or any upsetting experience from the past. It is best to pick something that still causes a little upset so you can experience how the treatment causes the upset to disappear.

If you wish to practice on family or friends, it is good to know that an important feature of TFT is the person guiding the treatment does not need any details or even need to know what specific trauma is being treated.

How to do the Trauma Algorithm

Step 1: Introducing the Treatment. TFT often appears strange,[2] unlike anything the person receiving the treatment has ever seen or heard before. Therefore we recommend you introduce the treatment by explaining you are experimenting with a new, risk-free procedure that is quite different and may seem a little strange. You might say something like this:

> "The TFT algorithm seems strange because it is not yet widely known. However, a very large number of therapists find it to be a safe and extremely powerful treatment. We can tell immediately whether it will help or not, since the effect is very rapid. We just need you to be as objective and accurate as you can when judging your emotions and reporting to us how you feel."

---

[2] I have a firm policy of requiring a new client to view the explanatory video, "Introduction to Thought Field Therapy." This one-hour video explains and demonstrates some of the basic principles of TFT and gives the client a context for its application.

Step 2: Tuning the Thought Field. Have the client think about the trauma and determine the degree of pain or discomfort on a scale of 1 to 10 (or a scale of 0 to 10) felt by the client when thinking about the trauma. This scale, often attributed to Dr. Joseph Wolpe, is known as the Subjective Units of Distress (SUD) Scale. Dr. Wolpe introduced the name.[3] Ask the client to rate the trauma, where 10 represents the worst upset possible and 1 represents no trace of upset. Record the SUD rating by writing it down in front of the client (see apex problem below). The more severe the upset, the more dramatic the demonstration.

You can say to the client: "Tell me, how uncomfortable you feel *at this moment,* thinking about the problem, on a scale from 1 to 10, where 10 is the worst you can feel and 1 is no trace of a problem. If we can reduce that upset now, that will be a good sign. If we can get the upset down to a 1, it is quite possible it will stay that way, but of course we won't know for sure until time passes."

Step 3: The Initial Treatment Sequence (the majors). The initial treatment sequence for trauma contains four treatment points:

---

[3] When I directed a U.S. Naval Research Project for Dean Eric Gardner (of Syracuse University Graduate School), and Professor George Thompson, they created a similar scale, prior to and independent of Dr. Wolpe, back in the early 1950s. I used this scale in 1949 and 1950 in my doctoral dissertation (Callahan, 1955). This highly sophisticated scale reflected the enormous skills of Dean Gardner, a top mathematician and statistician, and Professor Thompson, a top psychologist. The scale was also used in a drug study in which I participated (Graham, Rosenblum, and Callahan, 1958).

TREATMENT POINT #1: Ask the client to tap with two fingers, the beginning of the eyebrow above the bridge of his/her nose (see diagram, below) five good taps, firm enough to put a little energy into the system but *not nearly hard enough to hurt or bruise.*

TREATMENT POINT #2: Next, ask the client to tap under his/her eye about an inch below the bottom of the eyeball, at the bottom of the center of the bony orbit, high on the cheek. Tap solidly, but not nearly enough to hurt—about five taps.

TREATMENT POINT #3: Ask the client to tap solidly under his/her arm, about four inches directly below the armpit, five times. This point is level with the nipple in the male and about the center of the bra under the arm in the female.

TREATMENT POINT #4: Find the "collarbone point" in the following manner. Take two fingers of either hand and run them down the center of the throat to the top of the center collarbone notch. From this point go straight down one inch, and to the right one inch. Tap this point five times.

STEP 4: CHECKING THE SUD. At this time, ask how the client feels now. Ask for a second SUD rating. If the decrease is 2 or more points, continue with Step 5. If there was no change or the change was only one point, starting at a SUD of 7 or higher,[4] *correct the psychological reversal* (see section below for psychological reversal corrections),

---

4 At the higher range of SUD, i.e., 7 or above, a reported change of only one point is suspect and often indicates "positive thinking" or a hoped for, rather than an actual, change.

and repeat Step 3. If you started with a SUD below 7, a change of 1 point is acceptable to continue.

STEP 5: THE NINE GAMUT[5] TREATMENTS. To locate the gamut spot on the top back of the hand make a fist with the non-dominant[6] hand. This causes the large knuckles to stand out on the back of the hand. Place the index finger of dominant hand in the valley between the little finger and ring finger knuckles. Move the index finger about one inch back toward the wrist. This point is called the "gamut" point. Ask the client to tap the gamut spot on the top back of his/her hand (about three to five times per second) and continue tapping while going through the nine procedures as follows (tapping about five or six times for each of the nine gamut positions). It is crucial to tap the gamut spot *throughout* the nine steps.

1. Eyes open

2. Eyes closed

3. Open eyes and point them down and to the left

4. Point eyes down and to the right

5. Whirl eyes around in a circle in one direction

---

[5] Named for what I call the "gamut point" due to the literal gamut of treatments done off this point which was found through numerous empirical tests I carried out over a number of years.

[6] Which hand doesn't matter but most prefer to tap with dominant hand.

6. Whirl eyes around in opposite direction—rest eyes and

7. Hum a few notes of any tune (more than one note)

8. Count from one to five

9. Hum a few notes of a tune again

STEP 6: REPETITION OF THE INITIAL SEQUENCE (THE MAJORS). Repeat Step 3. After this repetition, thinking of the presenting problem will usually not bring any trace of an upset and hence be a 1 (or 0 if an 11-point SUD scale is used). If the SUD rating has decreased significantly, but is not yet a 1, have the client *correct mini-psychological reversal (mini-PR, see below) and repeat Steps 3-6.*

THE CALLAHAN TECHNIQUES™
TREATMENT POINTS

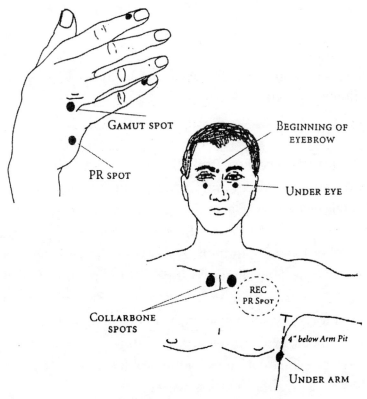

GAMUT SPOT

PR SPOT

BEGINNING OF EYEBROW

UNDER EYE

COLLARBONE SPOTS

REC PR SPOT

4" below Arm Pit

UNDER ARM

°1985 Dr. Roger J. Callahan • May not be reproduced
78816 Via Carmel • La Quinta, CA 92253

STEP 7: FLOOR-TO-CEILING EYE ROLL. The floor-to-ceiling eye roll is performed at the end of a successful series of treatments. When the client reports a 1 or 2 on the scale, this treatment serves to solidify a 1 and bring a 2 to a 1.

The client taps the gamut spot on the back of his/her hand while his/her head is held rather level (many people want to move their head in this exercise instead of their eyes). We use the word "rather" because some deviation from the level is acceptable. The client looks down, then slowly and steadily raises his/her eyes all the way up (taking about 10 seconds). The gamut spot *must* be tapped during the moving of the eyes. This exercise will typically bring a 2 down to a 1.

Psychological Reversal (PR)

Psychological reversal (PR) can prevent an otherwise successful treatment from working due, we believe, to a literal polarity reversal in the meridians.[7] To correct a PR, tap what we call a PR[8] spot, located on the outside edge of either hand about midway between the wrist and the base of the little finger. The PR spot is at the point of impact if one were to do a karate chop. PR is not a treatment for a psychological problem but rather a treatment for a block, which prevents a treatment from working; therefore, the treatments for the problem (Steps 2-6) *must be repeated* after the PR is corrected.[9]

---

[7] The "meridians" refers to the meridians of energy described in acupuncture and have been found to be quite palpable and supported by scientific investigation. The astonishing results of these treatments can be taken themselves as powerful evidence for the reality and specificity of these meridians.

[8] There are other PR correction procedures for different purposes, omitted for simplicity.

[9] The reversal correction will improve the success of *any* effective healing procedure.

If you correct psychological reversal before each treatment you will not get to observe the awesome PR effect. Some therapists like to begin every treatment with the automatic correction of psychological reversal, whether needed or not. It does no harm if a person is not reversed and the PR treatment is done. The correction of PR will not create a reversal. However, it is not advisable, as it prevents the therapist from observing the important phenomenon of psychological reversal. The change is usually very dramatic. A treatment which produced no change, will suddenly become effective (i.e., produce a drop of at least 2 points in the SUD) when that same previously ineffective treatment is repeated after the PR correction. If the person is not a professional it is not as important to experience the PR in action. It is quite acceptable for non-professionals to correct the PR whether or not it is needed.

Mini-Psychological Reversal (mini-PR) Correction

This is the procedure carried out when a client shows improvement, say from a 10 down to about a 3 or 4 but does not go lower. We call this a mini-PR problem, which is a polarity block that kicks in after a major improvement has taken place. Ask the client to tap the PR spot, as described above and repeat the entire treatment. Until the mini-PR was discovered, about three years after the PR, I had to frequently be satisfied with a treatment being partially effective. At the time the treatment was so dramatic, even though incomplete, both my clients and I were thrilled. Later, I wanted more improvement and wondered why some people went all the way down to a 1 while others stopped at a 3 or 4. I then discovered the mini-PR and its correction.

When a traumatized individual comes down from a high SUD score to a low, the treatment effect usually endures over time. Our clients are challenged to try to resurrect the upset. If any upset can be generated, the treatment is not finished. If any degree of upset occurs after the client leaves, I ask him/her to immediately call for another brief appointment and treatment. It is now easy, in our more advanced work, to re-treat or address another aspect of the problem. It is very important to discover through causal diagnosis exactly what caused the problem to return. I have mastered the issue of the rare return of a successfully treated problem.

PHOBIA TREATMENT

If you would like to help a person with a phobia, follow the treatment as indicated above, but substitute the following for the majors: Tap under eye (about an inch below the eyeball) five times. Remember to tap gently. Then tap under the arm (about four inches below the armpit) about five times. I use my fist for this one but that does not mean you pound it—just tap it gently five times. Then tap the point called the collarbone point five times. You then do the nine gamut procedure described above and then repeat the eye, arm, and collarbone treatment. The rules of correcting for psychological reversal are the same as when helping a trauma.

If the phobia treatment does not seem to help and you have done the PR correction, try this variation: Instead of starting with under the eye, start with under the arm, *then* tap under the eye, then the collarbone. The rest of the procedure is as above. Typically, this latter treatment works best for claustrophobia, and fear of spiders or turbulence while flying. The previous phobia treatment works best for all other phobias.

It is important to understand the difference between a phobia and anxiety disorder. A phobia is characterized by feeling fear only when in the presence of a feared situation or entity, whereas anxiety can hit at any time. People with anxiety are sometimes helped with the phobia treatments but are usually more complex than the simple algorithm. The treatment of choice for anxiety disorders is individualized help with a trained Callahan Techniques® TFT practitioner. Call our office for a referral.

When I worked with clients in person (today I treat everyone with the more powerful Voice Technology™ over the telephone) I had a sign in my office that stated in very large type: *"I CAN'T THINK ABOUT THE PROBLEM!"* Since the client had always gotten upset whenever the trauma was thought about prior to treatment, the person wrongly concludes that he or she must not be thinking about it if there is no upset. In small type the sign said. *"What I mean rather is that now, thanks to the effective treatment, I no longer get upset **when** I think about the problem."*

(Mark Steinberg, Ph.D., VT[10] has written a clever rap poem which features this interesting phenomenon. See Appendix, "I Just Can't Thought About it Anymore." The better you understand TFT the more you will appreciate this rap.)

THE TOOTH, SHOE, LUMP PRINCIPLE

In a small number of complex clients a complication may take place which I call the tooth, shoe, lump (TSL) principle. Here is an illustration of this principle. Consider a person who has a terrible toothache: He calls the dentist and rushes over to the office. Although there is no opening in the schedule, the dentist will take care of the problem as soon as she can. The tooth was hurting so much the patient had put on the first pair of shoes available, ignoring the fact these shoes hurt his feet. Due to the intense tooth pain, however, he doesn't notice the discomfort caused by the shoes.

When he gets to the office he sits on a couch directly upon a most uncomfortable lump. Again, this goes unnoticed due to the severe pain in the tooth. Just then the dentist comes out and indicates she will be able to attend to the problem in about an hour and a half, but seeing the severity of the pain, she injects a shot of Novocaine to give temporary relief. The tooth is suddenly relieved of all pain and the patient now becomes aware he put on the wrong shoes and is aware his feet are quite uncomfortable. He removes the shoes and in a moment he begins

---

[10] VT indicates that one is trained at the Voice Technology™ level, the highest level of TFT Causal Diagnosis.

to be aware of the uncomfortable lump upon which he has been sitting. He moves to a nearby chair and, at last, feels comfortable.

Something similar occurs in some severely complex clients who are only aware of a summation effect of their problems and do not, or are not able to, discriminate between say, trauma, anxiety and depression, or mixtures of various other problems. There can also be different aspects to one traumatic event that might need to be treated separately, if the person does not fully respond to treating the trauma as a whole, though the necessity for this is rare. The person being treated might not be aware of this. All he or she knows is he or she feels bad. We may completely remove all traces of the first problem in line, as confirmed by our tests and supported by the fact no complications such as PR or mini-PR show up on diagnosis. Often we are actually treating what the client may perceive as one problem but which may consist of a melange of problems.

IS IT DESIRABLE TO ELIMINATE ALL UPSET ASSOCIATED WITH A TRAUMA?

This question was a moot issue before there were powerful treatments to eliminate the bad effects of a trauma. I maintain it is desirable to eliminate all bad effects of a trauma. Some therapists who have learned how to do this work believe they should not eliminate all suffering, but leave some. They have the belief, quite wrong in my opinion, that leaving some measure of suffering will help protect the person against further trauma. I suspect this interesting notion became introduced through good treatments which were not completely effective and the residue that could not be eliminated was rationalized as a desirable situation. It is crucial to understand that, although TFT can eliminate all traces of a problem, *the treatment does not make a person stupid or ignorant.* I find a person can use more intelligence the less upset he or she is. This is the best protection one can have through treatment.

COMPLEX TRAUMA ALGORITHM

This treatment will eliminate all traces of a person's upset over a trauma anywhere in the range from 70-90% of the time. If you have followed the above instructions and you are unable to eliminate the upset, do not continue to repeat this treatment, as this will only result in unnecessary frustration. You may try the complex trauma algorithm.

After completing Steps 1-6 and any needed PR corrections, ask the client to tap the four treatment points for the complex trauma algorithm.

TREATMENT POINT #1: Have the client tap the inner tip of the little finger five taps (see diagram of hand)

TREATMENT POINT #2: Have the client tap the collarbone spot five times

TREATMENT POINT #3: Have the client tap the inside tip of the index finger (thumb side) five times

TREATMENT POINT #4: Have the client tap the collarbone spot five times.

CHECKING THE SUD. At this time, ask for another SUD rating or how the person feels now. If the decrease is 2 or more points, continue with the nine gamut procedures. If there was no change or the change was only one point if you started at a SUD of 7 or higher, *correct psychological reversal,* and repeat Treatment Points 1-4 of the complex trauma algorithm. If you started with a SUD below 7, a change of 1 point is acceptable to continue.

Ask the client to do the nine gamut procedures and then repeat the above Treatment Points 1-4. End the session with the floor-to-ceiling eye roll (as described in previous algorithm treatment sequence).

If you are unable to get results with this trauma algorithm, and you have corrected for PR, then it is necessary to see a professional trained in these procedures. A person properly trained in Callahan Techniques® TFT will be able to find the precise treatment sequence through causal diagnosis. Call our office for referrals to qualified practitioners.

CHAPTER 4

HOW TFT CAN HELP WITH DIFFERENT TYPES OF TRAUMA

A wide variety of experiences come under the heading of trauma. In this chapter, I will give a few of the many examples of how the TFT trauma algorithm has helped people with different traumatic experiences. You will learn how you can apply it to a wide variety of different types of trauma.

LOVE PAIN

Upset and loss from romantic rejection and disappointment, while not the most objectively horrible trauma, is often the most acutely painful to the person suffering. In my extensive therapy experience, I would say there is no more devastating emotional pain than romantic loss or rejection. There are many things objectively more terrible than romantic or love pain, but for depth and severity of reaction, love pain is right at the top. Many murders and suicides occur as a result of the devastating pain of lost romantic love. People experience such a loss as a rejection of who they are at the very core of their being and the hurt therefore goes very deep (Callahan, 1982).

These experiences happen not only to adults but to children and adolescents as well. Such experiences are typically not taken seriously by the adults around them and written off as "puppy love." However, these upsetting, often traumatic events may result in emotional devastation that is just as bad, if not worse, than it is for someone in a more mature relationship. Shakespeare's Juliet was only fourteen years old.

The pain and trauma suffered as a result of romantic loss can be enough to affect a person's ability as an adult to develop and sustain romantic relationships. Such people develop what I call amouraphobia, the fear of being devastated in a romantic relationship. These individuals are afraid to commit to intimate relationships because of the pain and hurt they suffered from earlier failed relationships. The worst part of this is that they are usually completely unaware of the role and power this fear has in sabotaging future successful romantic love relationships. I detailed the many manifestations and consequences of amouraphobia in my earlier book, *It Can Happen to You: The Practical Guide to Romantic Love*, which was a Book-of-the-Month Club selection. However, at the time this book was written, I was just beginning to develop treatments for amouraphobia and love pain. Use the trauma treatment in Chapter 3, to help heal yourself and/or your partner from past or present love pains.

ILLNESS OR THE ILLNESS OF A LOVED ONE

Having a serious chronic or terminal illness, or observing the same in a loved one, is very traumatic and stressful. As mentioned in the case of the terminally ill woman in an earlier chapter, TFT cannot change the fact of the illness, but it can relieve extreme emotional upset and stress due to the illness and greatly enhance the quality of life. Decreasing stress improves the chance for healing.

At a recent conference, I publicly treated an 82-year-old woman who had endured several years of living and caring for her husband who suffered from Alzheimer's disease, ending with his very slow and agonizing death. She had been with him at the time of his death and could not get the painful image out of her mind. Since her husband's death, which occurred years earlier, she had not been able to stop visibly shaking and was unable to think about anything else. I treated her in front of about fifty professionals at the behavioral medicine conference where I was demonstrating my discoveries.

She had come hoping that something might help her with this acute suffering. After one very brief treatment of about two minutes, she stopped visibly shaking and her upset was completely eliminated. She and the group were shocked and thrilled with the relative ease of treatment and the elimination of her suffering. In some cases where there is trauma that has occurred over a period of several years as in this example, more treatments might be necessary. You may need to treat each upsetting event or different aspect of the situation. Fortunately, multiple treatments were not necessary in this case.

JOB-RELATED STRESS AND TRAUMA

Whether a boss or an employee, there are many types of upsets and stresses that occur in connection with conditions of employment. The trauma treatment can help someone suffering from the trauma of being fired or laid off, as well as the many upsets that can occur during the course of a working day. One of the professionals I trained has specialized in consulting in the area of workplace violence and trauma. Large companies contract with him to treat employees who suffer from job-related upsets and problems including workplace violence, trauma and sexual harassment. TFT is very appealing to the businessperson because employees can be helped effectively and quickly. This simple but powerful treatment often results in increased harmony in the workplace and more productive employees.

People who have jobs where they have to deal with trauma, such as those in public service and disaster-relief organizations—including police officers, firemen, paramedics, doctors, nurses, and other hospital workers—are often themselves very traumatized by what they witness in their day-to-day work. Regular use of the trauma algorithm can help prevent burnout for the workers. It has also successfully helped the search-and-rescue dogs.

The TFT treatment for trauma is very effective in eliminating secondary trauma. One therapist I trained has worked in a hospital for twenty years and uses this treatment for herself on a daily basis. She reports that the treatment has helped her tremendously in dealing with the stress and upset she used to suffer as a result of what she is exposed to on the job.

CRIME VICTIMS

This treatment is tremendously effective for people who have been victimized by crimes. It has helped many people to eliminate the fear, distress and nightmares that result from such an experience. One of the many people I have helped was a fourteen-year-old girl who was shot in the leg as the result of a drive-by shooting. Her therapist was unable to help her and referred her to me. For eight months she had been traumatized and experienced nightmares due to the shooting. She couldn't get the frightening noise of the gunshots and the shattering glass out of her head. She suffered from nightmares in which she relived the shooting and would awaken terrified and very upset.

She came to me for help eight months after the shooting. When asked to think about the shooting she got very upset. The TFT treatment for trauma took less than ten minutes and removed all traces of her upset. The nightmares stopped. Even though this shooting was a horrible event, she was no longer upset or bothered by it and was free to go on with her life without having to relive the event, over and over. Five years after this treatment, the client reported that she remained free of all upset and the nightmares were gone.

CHILD ABUSE

People who have suffered multiple instances of abuse, such as repeated child abuse, can be helped with TFT. If you have suffered from this type of abuse and it is still affecting your life, the treatment given in this book will likely help. (Caution: Do not try the trauma algorithm on yourself if you are unable to even think about the event without severe, devastating upset. In that case, we recommend you call our office for a referral to a qualified therapist trained in these procedures who can work with you.)

Sometimes, in the case of complex, multiple traumas such as prolonged child abuse, the person will need more than one treatment. Multiple treatments may be needed in order to address the different traumas that occurred, and the gamut of feelings and disturbances connected with them.

Shirley's mother claimed that, five years before, when Shirley was three, she had been the victim of severe sexual and ritualistic abuse at her preschool. She also reported having been sexually abused in her home by a man with whom her mother used to live. Shirley had been in therapy for these traumas for five years with a traditional psychologist at a well-known medical center and had shown no noticeable improvement. She was still termed an elective mute. Talking about such an experience is, in and of itself, often re-traumatizing. As a result of her experiences, Shirley had nightmares and many fears. She was afraid of strangers, going into dark places, going to the bathroom alone, and going into certain rooms of her house. She also feared all kinds of windows because her abusers had told her she was being watched.

A friend in the law enforcement field referred her mother to me. Although very skeptical, she first came to see me for help with her own fear of public speaking. She wanted to test out the treatment herself before bringing in her daughter. Since I was able to quickly eliminate her fear of public speaking, she brought her daughter in to see me.

Shirley had two sessions with me. I treated her fears and upset one by one. Fortunately, when being treated with TFT, the client does not have to talk about or relive the upsetting experiences for the treatment to be effective. By the end of the first session, she was visibly more relaxed. When asked if she would like to come back to see me, she readily agreed, which she had not done in her previous therapy sessions. Her mother reported that after the first session she was able for the first time, to talk about what had happened to her. She became more comfortable around people and was able to go into rooms that she had been afraid to go into before the treatment. Shirley did so well she was able to stop seeing the therapist she had been seeing regularly for the past five years. She had one brief relapse, after the verdict was announced in the court case that set her alleged abusers free. This was quickly and successfully treated in one more very brief (minutes) session of TFT. She continues to do well.

Natural or Man-made Disasters

People who suffer the traumatic aftereffects of disasters such as hurricanes, earthquakes, floods, bombings, plane crashes and the wide array of other possible disasters, can benefit significantly from the TFT trauma algorithm. When we had a major earthquake in the Palm Springs area where we live, I successfully treated several people who had been severely traumatized. Prior to treatment they were living in constant fear of another earthquake.

One woman I treated had been in an earthquake in the Philippines over twenty years before. She still had nightmares about this frightening event. She now lived in Southern California and was in constant fear about the possibility of an earthquake occurring. The slightest rumble would send her into a panic. After I treated her and removed all traces of upset, nature provided us with a good test of the treatment. Three days later we experienced a minor earthquake and she showed no trace of fear. About a year later, she returned to the Philippines. Soon after her arrival a major earthquake occurred. She told me that during the entire earthquake, while other people were terrified and falling apart, she was able to remain calm and to be of assistance to other people who were panicking. Here was an acid test of the treatment.

Dr. Jenny Edwards, a marvelous and gifted therapist I trained in TFT, happened to be doing some therapy training in Nairobi, Kenya, at the time of the embassy bombing in August 1998. She went to the hospital and helped a number of the victims who had been injured and severely traumatized by this horrible event. The following is an excerpt from an article Dr. Edwards wrote for our newsletter, *The Thought Field:*

> I went up to a woman in the hospital lying on her bed, staring into space, and began talking with her. She was in a great deal of physical pain—a 10 on a 10-point scale, where this indicates that the pain is as bad as it can be. The bombing had blown off her shoes, and she had walked out of the embassy. As a result, she had a lot of glass in her feet, among other injuries, and was on strong pain medication but it didn't give much relief. Since her injuries weren't quite as severe as others, the doctors hadn't had a chance to work with her yet. After building rapport, I said timidly, "I have something that MIGHT help you. I'm not sure if it will work. It would involve tapping on these particular places on your body (I showed her), and would take about five minutes. I'm willing to try, if you would like me to."
>
> She said, "I'll do anything. I'm in so much pain. I also keep thinking that a bomb will explode any minute in the hospital. I know that it's probably not going to happen; however, I can't get the thought out of my mind!"
>
> I decided to work with the pain first. After tapping the pain algorithm, the SUD came down from a 10 to a 5; however, it wouldn't go any lower. It occurred to me that we needed to tap for trauma before the pain would go any lower. Of course, the trauma was a 10, and it came down to a 0 immediately after administering the trauma algorithm. After

that, we tapped again for pain, and it readily went down to a 0.

She blinked her eyes and looked at me, a little bewildered. She said, "I've played the pictures of what happened the day of the bombing over and over in my mind, almost without stopping, since Friday. It's really strange, but I'm not doing that any more. I think that I'll be able to get to sleep tonight." Then she looked straight at me, smiled, and said, "God saved me for a reason."

"Yes, He did," I said. I told her that the pain probably would return, and wrote out what she could do when it did. I told her that the trauma probably wouldn't return; however, if it did, the directions were there for her to follow.

About that time, the Sister came to me and said, "The woman in the bed across the way says she wants to be healed, too." I went over to her. She was just staring into space. Her arm was bandaged, and her hand was limp. After talking with her for a few minutes, I asked her if it would hurt if she tapped on the hand that was limp. She said it might hurt a little; however, it would be worth it in order to be able to experience the changes that she had just seen the woman in the bed across the way experience. She was 10 on both trauma and pain. I decided to work on trauma first. It came down fairly quickly to a 0, with no psychological reversal.

Then, we worked on the pain, which had already gone down to an 8 after working on the trauma. As she tapped, it went down to 0, too. She was moving her hand all around, color was restored to her face, and she was smiling and laughing. I wrote down what we had done. Her husband, who had been watching, asked the Sister if it might help his neck pain. She said, "Of course." By now, the first woman was sitting up for the first time since the bombing, eating dinner and talking with her husband. They were smiling and laughing. Her husband told the Sister that usually she panicked when it was time for him to leave at night because she didn't want to be alone, for fear a bomb might explode. He reported that this evening, for a change, she felt fine about his leaving, and told him that she would see him the next day. She then told the Sister that she had been on extremely high and frequent doses of pain medication, and was planning to use the tapping to lessen the amount and frequency of the doses.

This report provides a dramatic example of what is possible with the algorithms or simple recipes of TFT. Clearly, our treatment for trauma is helpful for a variety of different types of traumas and life upsets. These treatments are effective 80-90% of the time. Thanks to TFT, it is no longer necessary for someone to have to live with the devastating aftereffects of a trauma. As with all TFT treatments, you don't have to take our word for it. You can try this treatment for yourself.

CHAPTER 5

CAUSAL DIAGNOSIS

Genuine realities in themselves can be distinguished from (mere) appearances by their predictability.

Albert Einstein

[O]ur concepts may be inadequate or false and the only way we can test them is by encounter with objective fact at the level of the tangible world...

Arthur M. Young (1976)

W e call psychological problems, appropriately enough, "disorders." In an interview, theoretical physicist David Bohm said, "If there were no order in the disorder, then there would be no help possible." The TFT causal diagnostic procedure reveals the specific order in disorders and we find that when this causal order is translated into specific treatments, this order is "on line" with reality as indicated by the common repeatable and reproducible fact the symptoms and sequelae of the treated problem are gone. Joseph Ledoux puts forth his pessimistic indelibility principle for emotions due to the amygdala, that this part of the brain structure is the *fundamental* causal element of disturbing emotions (wrongly assumed, according to our robust evidence). The indelibility principle is a logical deduction since the amygdala is hardware rather than software. However, the information at a deeper software level, having less inertia than the hardware, is not recalcitrant and not indelible. Hence powerful and rapid psychological transformations are now not only possible but commonplace due to the more fundamental level of information revealed by the causal diagnosis procedures. Conventional psychotherapeutic treatments lend robust support to the indelibility hypothesis due to their ineffectiveness (Adler, Science Directorate Report, 1993; also see Rutter, 1994).

Diagnosis in psychology and psychiatry is nosological. A patient is placed into a descriptive category that best fits the predominant set of symptoms presented. The notion of *causal* diagnosis is, as far as I can determine, unknown to the field. In my almost half-century of practice, I have never heard of causal diagnosis in psychology. Callahan Techniques® Thought Field Therapy introduces the exciting new domain of causal diagnosis.

We posit that the fundamental causes of psychological problems are what we call perturbations (P's), which we further posit are localized within specific thought fields (Callahan and Callahan, 1996). Causal diagnosis means these fundamental causes are explicitly revealed in our diagnostic procedures, in their correct order (order is often crucial). Once the perturbations are revealed, the problem can be treated with unusual and unprecedented success. This is a profound advance.

ORDER IS VITAL

Please keep in mind that, for the majority of trauma victims, causal diagnosis is not required. Through my use of causal diagnosis, I was able to find a common algorithm or recipe that will help most people. Some naïve individuals found my algorithms so seemingly simple they quite wrongly proclaim that order is irrelevant. I will address this issue in much more detail in another book. The professionals who understand Voice Technology™ and who work with many more complex cases understand that in difficult and complex cases *order is as vital as it is in opening a combination lock.* It is not sufficient merely to have the right numbers for the code—they must be given in the proper order.

When the algorithm doesn't work for someone, we move up to causal diagnosis. When that doesn't work, then Voice Technology™ (the most accurate and refined causal diagnosis extant) is needed to help this complex problem.

A few uninformed individuals have assumed that randomly tapping the twelve different points will do as well as causal diagnosis. But I know from much experience in working with complex cases that the order the points are addressed is crucial. For years I have specialized in significantly helping clients that my diagnostically trained and highly competent professionals were unable to help. I have had more experience in helping complex problems than any therapist in history.[1] Keep in mind that even with complex cases, the treatment is rapid (perhaps an hour or two). Let us calculate the odds of coming up with the correct order for a treatment sequence in a complex case by randomly tapping. The odds of finding the correct order for treating a complex problem[2] by random tapping on points can be calculated by finding 12 factorial (i.e., 12 x 11 x 10 x 9 x 8 and so on). Twelve factorial tells us there are 479,001,600 possible combinations of 12 different points. If it took only one minute to apply five taps to each of the twelve points it would take 911 years to carry out all combinations. That is, if one only tapped and did not sleep, eat, work or anything else 24 hours each day. This calculation is conservative because it leaves out the nine gamut and the psychological reversal corrections, as well as other treatments.

This calculation is for one series of treatments. Some complex clients need two, three or even as many as fifty or more series. For two correct series in a row it would take 10 to the 25th power seconds if done by chance.

---

[1] This record is certain to be surpassed in the future by the younger professionals whom I have trained in Voice Technology™.

[2] I established two decades ago that some individuals can be cured by addressing just *one* meridian. However, to increase the success rate, I had to find additional effective treatments. It is easy to understand that some easily treated individuals could mislead some naïve practitioners into missing the point regarding the need for causal diagnosis in complex cases.

One can get an idea for the tremendous size of this number by looking at the number of seconds since the universe started,[3] i.e., since the time of the Big Bang. The answer is 10 to the 18th power (Foster, p. 83). This means that finding the correct treatments for very complex clients would be impossible[4] without the development of causal diagnosis. It is no wonder these solutions were not discovered before I developed causal diagnosis.

Success Rate

In order to appreciate the following argument it is necessary to be aware of the extraordinarily high success rate of TFT. For example, a number of years ago, soon after Voice Technology™ (VT) was developed, I treated, in public, a group (N=68) of skeptical strangers with a success rate of 97% (see Table 1 for details). VT has the highest success rate.

Success Rate and Prediction

Keep in mind our high success rate, which takes place in minutes, is a scientific prediction. More than that, it is a prediction that is shocking; it is a prediction that goes against all conventional knowledge; it is a radical prediction. The prediction level with TFT algorithms is close to that of hard science (physics and chemistry); the prediction level with Voice Technology™ is easily on a par with

---

[3] Please note: The time the *universe* started; the earth came much later.

[4] Foster explains (p. 81) that physicists have defined "never" and "impossible" in terms of "zero in any operational sense of an event."

hard science. Prediction is exciting in science for it is a test of the relationship of our ideas to reality. When our predictions are correct, we know we are "on line" with reality.

> *We can predict things...for a theoretical physicist the greatest experience is to predict some things, to find that predictions work and thus to demonstrate the confluence between human thought and nature.*
>
> Ilya Prigonine
> Nobel Laureate

TABLE 1

**Telephone Treatment of Individuals Suffering
From Phobias and Anxiety on Call-In Radio Shows:
The Callahan Study, and a replication,
ten years later, by Leonoff**

(Causal Diagnoses performed with Voice Technology™)

	Original (1985-6)	VT Trainee (1995)
Number of radio shows	23	36
Number treated	**68***	**68**
Successful	66	66
Unsuccessful	2	2
Success Rate	97%	97%
Average SUD (pre-therapy)	**8.35** (10-point scale)	**8.19** (11-point scale)
Average SUD (post-therapy)	**2.10** (1=best possible)	**1.58** (0=best)
Average Time (minutes—Includes all explanation to the end of treatment)	**4.34**	**6.04**

*In Callahan's study a breakdown was done to provide a measure of the effect of treatment in an actual exposure situation. In talking on the radio the individuals were engaged in public speaking. Fear of public speaking is the most common fear, and **11** subjects treated in this study suffered from this fear. The average SUD before treatment = **8.8;** after treatment = **1.9**. The average time for this sub-group, including description of the problem, diagnosis, and explaining the unfamiliar treatment, was **5.16 minutes**. All 11 of the subjects were

helped dramatically in this reality test of the treatment. The high success rate of this small sub-sample does not imply that the brief treatment will cure everyone of this common phobia; if the N were higher
for this sub-group, some failure could be counted upon, especially
within the time constraints of radio shows.

To minimize selective bias in the analysis of results, *all* people who
called in were treated, including those individuals whose treatments
were cut short due to time constraints; all were included in these
analyses. As in the earlier study, audiotapes of all treatments were
made and are available for review.

A decade later, the study was independently replicated by a VT trainee, Leonoff, with close to identical results (N also = 68—see same Table 1 above).

In the November 1998 TFT newsletter, Dr. Stephen
Daniel reports still another VT clinical study. Using VT, he
treated 214 therapists who presented problems that did
not respond to other therapy procedures, including the
ordinarily effective TFT algorithms. This group had an average pre-therapy SUD (Subjective Units of Distress) of
7.74 and an average post-therapy SUD of 1.11 (where 1
indicates no distress or pain at all). The average time for
diagnosis and treatment per person was 4.98 minutes.
The success rate is comparable to the previous two independent clinical studies. (For those who may be dubious
about SUD, we have internal checks which help assure us
of the accuracy of reported SUD, we also have profound
laboratory scientific evidence of the deep biological effects of these treatments. Personally, I believe that there
is no substitute for SUD.)

Following is a brief report from Monica Pignotti,
LCSW, that I recently received on an additional survey of
treatment success with VT. These treatments were per-

formed at various algorithm trainings after available methods had not helped.

> Total people treated = 72
> Pre-Treatment SUD = 7.83
> Post-Treatment SUD = 1.05
> Success Rate = 98.5%

A recent clinical report from Ian Graham of the United Kingdom reports a success rate of 94% in treating 177 individuals over a six-month period using the middle level of success, the Callahan Techniques® TFT (CTTFT) Causal Diagnostic procedures. Eleven individuals did not respond to the treatments in this study. The pre-treatment average SUD was 8.29 and the post treatment average SUD 2.17.

The total number of individuals included in these five (four with VT and one with causal diagnosis) independent success rate reports is **594.** The success results are all extremely high and quite predictable with this approach. Professionals who know how to do CTTFT are usually willing to treat skeptical strangers in public. If they did not have confidence there was a good chance for success, they would not be so willing to engage in this professionally risky procedure. Because of these results, we can make strong predictions due to the accuracy of the causal diagnoses and the resulting power of this therapy. The high predictability of this work establishes it closer to hard science than the soft science so common to psychology.

An Upper Limit on Possible Treatment Success

Can any treatment be 100% successful? I don't believe so. I have often said that anyone who reports a 100% success rate either has a selective memory or simply has not treated enough clients. Bohm (1957, p. 143) in speaking of hard science (not psychotherapy) says: "Actually, however, neither causal laws or laws of chance can ever be perfectly correct because each inevitably leaves out some aspect of what is happening in broader contexts." Considering that Bohm is referring to hard science, it is not a huge jump to figure that our already high treatment success must be pushing very close to perfection. Of course, we in CTTFT do not, and will not, stop trying to improve the success of our work.

> *The pursuit of truth will set you free—even if you never catch up to it.*
>
> Clarence Darrow

Continuing Increases in Success Rate

An important factor in grasping the causal nature of TFT diagnostic procedures is that at the time of the first discovery in Callahan Techniques® (curing a severe water phobia, about two decades ago), my success rate was in the neighborhood of 3%. Through the causal diagnostic procedures, which I gradually developed and honed over time, the success rate today has grown to 97-99+%.[5] It is clear that an improvement in the success rate of this unprecedented magnitude is likely to be addressing the fundamental causal elements of the problem.

When this work began, about 20 years ago, I was naturally the only one reporting high success. However, as more professionals learned to do the procedures they, too, reported unprecedented success. There are now many thousands throughout the world who are duplicating my results. The almost perfect VT results are due to numerous discoveries I made and they clearly demonstrate that the VT procedure is teachable and the high results reproducible. (This fact itself has important scientific implications. See for example, Cowen, who in 1999 reported a planetary system found in outer space—a surprising finding and a first of its kind. Three groups of astronomers worked on this: one from Harvard-Smithsonian Center for Astrophysics in Cambridge, Mass.; another at the Anglo-Australian Observatory; and another at San Francisco State University and University of California-Berkeley. Note the wording that Peter Nisenson of Harvard uses: "By having two independent [data] sets, we're just extremely positive that this is all real.")

About such an increase in success, Bohm (who, as far as I can determine, has written more exhaustively on causality in science than any one else) states: "...scientific research does not and cannot lead to a knowledge of

---

[5] Within the last year I have made two new discoveries in Voice Technology™ which have added to the already high success rate. While in Japan in July 1999, I made an additional discovery.

nature that is completely free from error. Rather it leads and is able to lead only to an unending process in which the degree of truth in our knowledge is continually increasing." This is an accurate description of my success rate, which started at about 3% twenty years ago and through a continuing process of discovery now is approaching (with VT) 99+%.

OTHER EVIDENCE

Obsessions and nightmares are common symptoms of post traumatic stress disorder. When we treat trauma we measure the pain, hurt and upset which accompanies this problem. In almost every instance we quickly eradicate the overwhelming disturbing symptoms. What is interesting, however, is that the nightmares and obsessions, which are not directly addressed, are also typically stopped with our trauma treatment. If the treatment were not in touch with the fundamental causal elements, improvements in these related aspects of trauma would be most unlikely.

RESPONSE TO TREATMENT PROPORTIONAL TO THE STAGES OF TREATMENT

The group data in Table I does not show the responses of the individual to various stages of the treatment—remember improvement is taking place within minutes, but nevertheless the changes predictably were related to the amount of treatment. There is a very clear and common pattern of response to the treatments such that the degree of response of the client is directly related to the amount of the treatment given (all of this, of course is within minutes, rather than days, weeks, months, or years,[6] and is predicted in advance). When you do the treatment for trauma included in this book, you will be able to observe this clear, predictable progress simply by asking the person to report how he or she feels after each of the steps of treatment. This will make the predicted progress clear. That the result is directly proportional to the treatment has basic scientific relevance.

The clients know nothing of psychological reversal (PR) and its profound effect completely blocking treatment. Nevertheless, they respond robustly in the predicted fashion when the PR treatment is given. The model for observing the PR effect is when a person does not respond to treatment. When the very same treatment is repeated after the reversal correction is given, *the PR treatment takes but 15 seconds!* It can clearly be observed that the very same treatment that a moment before did nothing suddenly results in a dramatic reduction of the problem.

This model of the PR effect is a very robust prediction and it is highly relevant that the treated person does not know what is supposed to happen, but nevertheless responds in the predicted fashion. This commonplace result lends further robust evidence of the objective value

---

[6] When treatment effects take place immediately, one must be prepared to acknowledge the effect of that treatment as the *cause* of change. If treatment spans months or years, this allows plenty of time for the operation of extraneous factors such as chance events or natural healing which have nothing whatsoever to do with the treatment given.

of these treatments. We estimate our treatments would be 40 to 50% less successful if we did not know how to correct for PR.

PREDICTIONS COMPARABLE TO HARD SCIENCE

If you recall high school or college science laboratory experiments, you will remember the predictions in hard science (e.g., physics and chemistry) are strong, but they are not perfect. Even carefully repeated scientific measures of gravity have produced slightly different results with each measurement.

Scientific laws are idealized in science; it was Galileo's genius to idealize rather than use exact results. David Peat (1987) said, "Laws of nature work exactly only in the imagined laboratories of physicists' minds" (p. 49). The law of gravity, for example, states that an apple accelerates 32 feet per second per second. (That is, each second the apple's speed is increased by an additional 32 feet per second.) How can it be determined to an arbitrary accuracy?

Peat spoke to Canadian scientists at the National Research Council of Canada who attempted such a measurement on a falling iron bar. "In trying to separate the experiment from the rest of the universe many hundreds of person-hours were used (e.g., evacuating the tube used for the fall; shielding to eliminate all electric and magnetic forces; temperature control to eliminate changes in expansion and contraction; timing done with atomic clock, and earth tremors were monitored. Extreme care was given to the way the bar was released—it had to be carefully controlled, one side released the tiniest fraction of a second before the other might start oscillation."

Even with all this, *each measurement differed slightly in its result.* The final value was obtained by averaging. But after all these controls, the averages over two separate series of measurements were "still different to a significant degree." It was concluded that *one couldn't isolate the universe effect completely.*

ELECTRICAL ENGINEERING LABORATORY PREDICTIONS

Compare the predictions of CTTFT Voice Technology™ in treating some problems of the mind with the predictions in experiments carried out in electrical engineering laboratories. For example, "...one of the experiments asks students to compare theoretical calculations with in-lab measurements on a real, operational oscillator. These comparisons [between theory and fact] routinely *agree to within a few percent* [my emphasis]." (Nahin, p. 141)

A few percent! What is a few percent? Anywhere from 2 to 4 percent error would result in 96 to 98% success rate. Actually from my recollection of high school and college science experiments in physics and chemistry, a few percent error would be considered excellent. Compare this error or failure rate with the success rate of TFT treatments—in treating real problems of the mind![7]

---

[7] Many experts consider the mind the most complex entity in the known universe. This presumed fact is often used as an explanation for the generally poor results in psychotherapy.

THEORETICAL PREDICTIONS WITH TFT CAUSAL DIAGNOSES

It is well known that psychological science makes no hard predictions, except perhaps negative ones such as the American Psychological Association's Science Directorate taking the position that phobias can *not* be cured. (Adler, 1993) Using my discoveries, even children are proving that this position (as well as that of LeDoux) is a serious error. (Daniel, 1997)

For example, Plotkin and Odling-Smee, in what might be considered an understatement, put the issue for conventional psychology clearly: "It is an old and often repeated lament that behavioral science at large is deficient in theory, and that what passes for theory is usually no more than a set of loosely articulated, incomplete, descriptive statements that make *no strong predictions* [my emphasis]." (In support, the authors cite several psychologists: Estes, Koch, MacCorquodale, Meehl, Mueller, Schoenfeld, Verplank, and Madsen.)

Many critics have taken psychological research on psychotherapy to task because the use of the term from statistics called "significance" gives a false impression. The use of this term implies that the results of a research study which shows "statistical significance" conveys *clinical* significance when no such relevant significance has been shown. Any minuscule difference between a control and an experimental group will be "statistically significant" as long as the groups are large enough. The clinical relevance is still another matter and conventional psychotherapy is woefully inadequate compared to the hard science of TFT.

One physicist once commented, "If you need to do statistics on your research study you should do a different study."

To compare our predictions in TFT with hard science predictions, we will consider our theoretical basis to be the diagnosed perturbations (which dictate the actual treatments given and their proper order). The real measurement equivalents are the resulting predicted reductions in the presenting problem as the specifically identified perturbations are addressed in treatment. We have four independent clinical experiments of causal diagnosed treatments with 527 people, as previously noted. In them, our success rates are comparable to those of hard science.

More important than these astonishing results themselves is the fact that perhaps no psychologists or psychotherapists would imagine such success rates would be possible in the field of psychotherapy. To put it mildly, TFT is counter-intuitive! No scientist would expect such results possible in the field of psychology, let alone in the more precarious field of psychotherapy where psychological problems are being addressed. This causal diagnostic work is a new domain of exciting science—to find discoveries, which no one would have thought possible—this is Callahan Techniques® Thought Field Therapy!

To those who believe this approach appears too simple, note what Karl Popper (1997), the most highly regarded philosopher of science, stated along these lines: "Science may be described as the art of systematic over-simplification." He also said, "What we want in science are bold ideas, controversial ideas, a solution to a problem."

His primary point was: "But with all respect for the lesser scientists, I wish to convey here a heroic and romantic idea of science and its workers: men who humbly devoted themselves to the search for truth, to the growth of our knowledge; men whose life consisted in an adventure of bold ideas. I am prepared to consider with them many of their less brilliant helpers who were equally devoted to the search for truth—for great truth. But I do not count among them those for whom science is no more than a profession, a technique: those who are not deeply moved by great problems and by the oversimplifications of bold solutions. It is science in this heroic sense that I wish to study." (p. 42)

He goes on to say that he does not attempt to define science, but only wishes to draw a "simple picture of the kind of men I have in mind, and their activities.... But it is not the present acceptance of the theory which I wish to discuss, but its boldness. *It was bold because it clashed with all then accepted views and with the prima facie evidence of the senses. It was bold because it postulated a hitherto unknown hidden reality behind the appearances* [my emphasis]." (p. 43)

Popper could have been writing about CTTFT, though it wasn't yet discovered. "It is the boldness of a conjecture which takes a real risk—the risk of being tested, and refuted; the risk of clashing with reality." (p. 46)

CAUSALITY IN GENERAL

How do we know fundamental causality in science? In general, we know causality due to high predictive success, especially when this success is unexpected or what is called "non-intuitive." We also can grasp causality when ministrations in a hitherto unknown area result in profound and predictable changes never before possible.

In their reply to the postmodern intellectuals' anti-scientific attitude, theoretical physicists Sokal and Bricmont point out that "the unexpected phenomenon often constitute the most spectacular tests of the validity of scientific ideas." (p. 68)

Here is a very concise statement that presents the scientific notion of causality: "The most practical and the only foolproof method of scientifically testing a causal connection between A and B is 'wiggling' one of them and watching the response of the other. We are...interested here in...'scientific causality' (establishing such a connection in repeatable events).... It is the external control of A together with the correlation with B that establishes...the causal connection between them, as well as the fact that A is the cause and B, the effect." (Newton, 1970)

David Bohm, in his thorough book on scientific causality (1957), states:

> An important way of obtaining evidence in favor of the assumption that a given set of events or conditions comes necessarily (i.e., is not a mere association) from another is to show that a wide range of changes in one or more of the presumed causes occurring under conditions in which other factors

are held constant always produces corresponding changes in the effects. The more coordinations of this kind that one can demonstrate in the changes of the two sets of events, the stronger is the evidence that they are causally related; and with a large enough number one becomes, for practical purposes, certain that this hypotheses of causal connection is correct.

A leading authority in the philosophy of mind is John Searle. Here are some comments on causality taken from his book (1997):

> Once we know two things are correlated, we still have not explained the correlation. Think of lightning and thunder, for example—a perfect correlation but not an explanation until we have a theory. Well, typically the next step in the sciences is to try and discover whether or not the correlation is a causal relation. Sometimes two phenomena can be correlated because they both have the same cause. Measles spots and high fever are correlated because they are both caused by a virus....

> One way to try and figure out whether the correlates are causally related to each other is to try to manipulate one variable and see what happens to the other....

> If you can manipulate one term by manipulating the other, then other things being equal, you have good evidence that the term you are manipulating is the

cause of the term manipulated, which is its effect.
(pp. 196-197)

Our two variables in CTTFT, of course, are 1) the perturbations in the thought field, which we propose are the fundamental cause of any disturbing emotion and which are revealed by causal diagnosis; and 2) the points on the body that I have discovered to be isomorphic to the specific perturbations in the thought field. We have overwhelming evidence to support this notion of isomorphism.

With our simple algorithms, it is quite easy for anyone to check out this causal isomorphic relationship. Algorithms (discovered through causal diagnosis and found to be successful for a high number of people), though highly successful in their own right, are not as successful as treatments derived from causal diagnosis. The difference in an algorithm and causal diagnosis is comparable to buying a man's suit off the rack vs. having the suit tailor-made to the individual's particular specifications. However, all my algorithms were originally discovered due to causal diagnosis.

Placebo

The term placebo means literally "I shall please." It comes from physicians who have no treatment for a particular problem and give an inert pill—a sugar pill. When the patient ascribes getting better to the pill, the result is called a "placebo effect." Presumably placebos are effective to the degree that the patient and/or the doctor "believe" in the power of the treatment.

When I first developed these treatments, I heard the placebo effect charge rather frequently; I still hear it today. In my first training of psychotherapists, I selected a militant skeptic to be the therapist, who would use my strange-seeming (non-intuitive) algorithm for phobias, and a militant skeptic who volunteered to have his intense phobia treated. It is, of course, quite natural to be skeptical of these procedures since they appear so strange to the unaccustomed eye. The treatment progressed as usual by predictably reducing the skeptical volunteer's intense phobia, and by the end of the brief procedure (a matter of minutes) the problem was completely gone. The strong disbelief, in both the therapist and the client, had no negative effect. The treatment is so powerful that it typically overcomes all negative resistance in reducing or eliminating the problem of non-believers. The skeptic therapist cured the skeptic client's phobia in less than five minutes! Most of the people who have taken my training were initially skeptical until they saw for themselves the powerful and unprecedented results of my treatments.

It is common that professionals will observe our dramatic results and then take the position these dramatic results are due to placebo effect. Never mind that in their whole career none of them have ever observed a placebo effect have such a dramatic predicted effect on so many people (and on young children, infants, dogs, cats, and horses).

Specialized medical experts in the philosophy of treatment have reviewed the standard research on placebo and have concluded that most of it is a total myth—they conclude that *there is no placebo effect* (Kienle and Kiene, 1996). The research on placebo, they found, is loaded with errors and misinterpretations. (The authors are physicians who are engaged in the epistemological and methodological bases of medicine, and are based at the Institute for Applied Epistemology and Medical Methodology in Freiburg, Germany. This work is a must-read for anyone in the healing arts.) They found the placebo illusion caused by spontaneous healing or improvement; symptom fluctuation; regression to the mean; additional treatment; scaling bias; irrelevant response variables; polite response; experimental subordination; conditioned answers; neurotic or psychotic misjudgment; psychosomatic phenomena; and misquotation. *In analysis of 800 publications on placebo, the authors state there were no valid demonstration of true placebo effects.*

It is common for professionals who observe an effective treatment with which they are unfamiliar to label the treatment "placebo." Placebo treatment might be called "someone else's treatment that has a positive effect."

How Long Does the Treatment Last?

Interestingly, in my thirty years of psychotherapeutic practice prior to my present discoveries, not once did anyone ever ask me the question after therapy, "How long will it last?" There was nothing palpable or demonstrable to last. Nothing dramatic happened when I did the conventional psychotherapies. I now hear that question frequently.

The endurance of therapy is, of course, a highly relevant question, but we have made another major breakthrough discovery that provides an unanticipated solution for a treatment that does not endure over time. I found that for the small number of people whose problem returns after a successful treatment, this return is due to an exogenous factor which can now be identified and eliminated. Once eliminated, and the problem is treated again (usually taking only a matter of minutes), the problem remains gone. In fact, with the ongoing research in this domain (to be the subject of a new book), we are able to predict and control the return of a problem that had been completely cured.

These discoveries have made psychotherapy a highly predictable and reliable method of treatment that goes far beyond one's greatest expectations. I can say that, after almost a half century of doing psychotherapy, it has now become a joyful enterprise! It is thrilling to be able to help so many people dramatically in so little time.

Keep in mind these findings, as strange and unexpected as they may seem, *can all be replicated by anyone who learns the proper procedures.*

CHAPTER 6

PSYCHOLOGICAL REVERSAL (PR)

"We have met the enemy and he is us."

Pogo (by Walt Kelly)

WHAT IS PSYCHOLOGICAL REVERSAL?

Psychological reversal (PR) is perhaps the most important single fundamental dynamic concept for health, human progress, happiness, and success that one may ever encounter. It is easy to learn how to treat for PR and to understand it. We also find it is easy to take it for granted and to lose sight of its dynamic import for natural healing and for psychological treatment. If it were not for the discovery of PR, the success rate of TFT would be reduced by as much as 40 to 50%. Many people today who are quickly cured of intense psychological problems would be completely untreatable if we did not understand and know how to correct the important but seemingly simple phenomenon of psychological reversal.

Psychological reversal was the first discovery I made among the numerous discoveries that constitute TFT. I identified it as a real phenomenon before I found a way to treat it. Not until a number of months later, after intensive searching and clinical research, did I discover a therapy for correcting PR. Prior to that, it was clear that PR was an undesirable state, associated with chronic problems. It carried with it a disposition toward destructive and self-destructive behavior.

Psychological reversal is a state of being which is caused by a simple polarity reversal within a system.[1] All of us at times can be and are in this state. When we are in a bad, destructive mood, this is almost always a sign that the PR state predominates.

When a new discovery is made, it is difficult to select a name for it that will likely endure into the unknown future. The term "psychological reversal" was first chosen because the state appeared to reverse the usual motivational state of the person. It appeared to turn the person against self-interest and toward self-defeat. I first viewed PR as a system that resulted in stress if the person wished to do good and no stress if harm or a self-destructive path was followed. This would be an obvious perversion within a system. The term PR was first viewed as a metaphor. Years later it was exciting to discover that the term is much

---

[1] The body/mind contains many systems and PR typically is specialized within a system of systems.

more than just a metaphor and actually refers to a concrete, literal reversal of polarity. During the state of PR there is a literal reversal of polarity involved. Harold Saxton Burr of Yale measured literal polarity in living things with a special voltmeter (Burr, 1972). He points out that every cell is polarized and that the sperm polarizes the egg.

Once one grasps the fact of a literal reversal, I am sometimes asked, "Since the PR is literally a polarity block in a particular system, why do you still use the term 'psychological,' why not just 'reversal'?" This is a sophisticated question, but the psychological part is an intrinsic factor when we wish to diagnose and or treat the PR. Having the person think of the problem is absolutely crucial in both diagnosis and in treatment. Tuning the problem is, of course, a psychological process and is an essential element in both the diagnosis and the treatment of the condition.

TYPES OF PR

Specific PR is the most common form and is limited to a specific area or areas of a person's life. For instance, a person who has a mental block to learning computers might be reversed only in the area of computers. This condition will make him appear inadequate in this one domain while in other pursuits he may be quite accomplished.

Massive PR is a reversal that affects most of a person's entire life, rather than just one specific area. A person who is massively reversed needs to be treated for this condition in order for any treatment to work. Such people are often in a chronic bad mood and exhibit a negative attitude towards life. (I have found that not *all* systems are reversed even in what I call a massive PR, just most or many.)

Mini-PR (MPR) occurs when a treatment is partially, but not completely successful. For example, in doing the trauma treatment, the person's level of upset goes from a SUD of 9 to a 4, but does not go any lower (without PR treatment).

Recurring PR is a psychological reversal that tends to return as soon as it is corrected. We have found this is most often due to toxins.

Behavioral Signs That Reveal PR is Present

Here are some common signs in everyday life that a PR is present:

Client shows no improvement after a usually effective treatment is administered. PR is corrected and then dramatic improvement takes place after a repeat of the very same treatment that *a moment prior to the PR correction did absolutely nothing*. This is a highly robust, predictable observation and will be easily observable if you refrain from correcting PR routinely prior to treatment.

Person reverses (or transposes) the correct order of letters or numbers. This effect is so commonplace that proofreaders have a special sign to indicate it. Whenever I find this or any other signs of PR in myself, I immediately correct my PR.

Person reverses directional concepts when in the PR state. For example, he will say "up" when meaning "down," or "right" when meaning "left," "north" when "south" is intended. (Interestingly, they will not say "west" or "east" when they mean "north," but only the opposite, "south.") Actions can be reversed also when in the PR state; for example, a person puts a cooked turkey in the oven instead of the intended refrigerator, or vice-versa. I find these reversals, correlated as they are to what I call PR, to be most interesting from a theoretical standpoint.

SOME EXAMPLES OF QUOTATIONS THAT FEATURE SOME ASPECT OF WHAT I CALL PR

The phenomenon of psychological reversal can be readily inferred as expressed in the following quotes:

> *Did you ever feel that life is an obstacle course and you are the biggest obstacle?*

> Jack Paar
> Original Tonight Show host

> *It's a pleasure to be here on the Larry Queen show.*[2]

> Jerry Spence, defense attorney
> Guest host on the Larry *King* show

> *For the good that I would I do not: but the evil which I would not, that I do....*

> *I find then a law, that, when I would do good, evil is present with me.*

---

[2] As is usual with PR, Spence showed no awareness that he had made this mistake.

For I delight in the law of God after the inward man:

But I see another law in my members, warring against the law of my mind, and bringing me into captivity to the law of sin which is in my members.

Saint Paul, Romans 7:18, 20, 22-23

An Incident of a Child's PR

A beautiful young four-year-old girl we shall call Judy had spent a long day with her parents riding on a boat, mixing and playing with a number of older relatives. Unexplainably, she suddenly began crying intensely, kicking and screaming. Surprisingly, nothing seemed to be able to relieve Judy's apparent agony, not to mention the agony of everyone in her presence.

Her mother reported that Judy had been screaming and carrying on for almost a straight hour, for no known reason. Mother looked over at me and asked, "Is there anything I can do?" I suggested that she do the simple PR treatment. With nothing to lose, her mother gently tapped the side of her hand used for the PR treatment and Judy suddenly became transformed. She abruptly stopped crying and began observing her surroundings and interacting with the dozen or so people present in the large summer cottage living room.

PR as a Block to Healing

The following is typical of the kinds of stories we hear all the time. I received a letter from Dr. John T. Hughes of

Ashland, Kentucky, a chiropractor and member of the International College of Applied Kinesiology. Dr. Hughes stated that in the 1980s, he was teaching a class of doctors and wanted to show them the phenomenon of PR he learned from an article I had written (Callahan, 1981b). He used the TFT diagnostic procedure for PR with a volunteer, a wife of one of the doctors.

The diagnostic test for massive reversal showed that she had no reversal (see Callahan Techniques® Causal Diagnosis Home Study Course). Her husband, who had heard of my notion of PR, asked Dr. Hughes to test her specifically about her jaw. Dr. Hughes then checked for specific reversal on her jaw by having her say: "I want my jaw to be healthy." She then showed she had a specific reversal that was mainly responsible for preventing an infection from healing. She had had a root canal performed on one of her teeth and developed a hole in her lower right jaw. This had continued to produce an exudate of pus for about a year and a half. She consulted another dentist, but the condition continued for they did not know why she didn't heal. Dr. Hughes then used my simple procedure for correcting reversal.

The treatment for PR occurred on a weekend and Dr. Hughes saw the doctor and his wife the following Thursday at a meeting. The doctor said, "I want to tell you what happened to my wife after you corrected her PR. That very evening the hole in her jaw really started to run and produce more exudate than ever before. Then it just stopped. They had the dentist examine the area and he said all the tissue appeared clear and healthy."

Dr. Hughes saw the couple a few months later and she said, "Do you want to see my scar?" The jaw was totally healed. This story fits many experiences of many doctors. A PR can prevent normal healing and the simple correction can often bring about dramatic changes.

One time I was flying home from the East Coast and I fell asleep with my right arm in a peculiar position. I awakened and the fingers in my right hand were all cramped. Rubbing the hand and arm and waiting for a time did nothing for this recalcitrant cramp. I tapped the PR point on the side of the hand, and immediately the fingers all relaxed and went to normal.

FRACTURES

It is well known among those who work in the field of orthopedics that a person may break a leg and, in a small number of cases, the fracture will not heal. This is quite serious, for the unhealed leg may need to be surgically removed. Interestingly, experienced orthopedic surgeons will sometimes put a battery or a magnet on the site of the fracture and, in some cases, this will result in healing. When this works it would seem the battery or magnet does something that corrects the literal polarity reversal in the healing system associated with the fractured leg (see Robert O. Becker; and Basset, Pawluk, and Pila; and also Nordenstrom).

My theory is that a psychological reversal is responsible for the lack of healing just as in the case of the jaw, and of course this is an easily testable notion. The PR treatment takes but seconds as you will see, and it would be easy to check out this theory. If the leg still does not begin healing immediately then we suggest a diagnostically trained TFT therapist be brought in to investigate why the PR was not correctable, which is a rare event but has a known cause for one properly trained in TFT. Often, in such cases, a knowledgeable TFT therapist can find the precise reason for the difficulty and, once found, the PR can usually be corrected.

A young man recovering from a severe case of paranoia for which he had been hospitalized is a member of a therapy group. Whenever he was psychologically reversed, it was obvious to all present from the expression on his face—this is not true of most people. When it is obvious, it is like neon sign reading "I am psychologically reversed!" Members of the group would immediately urge him to correct his PR. The moment he did this, his face changed dramatically.

EVIDENCE FOR PR

In addition to the observations noted above, there are a number of different types of evidence supporting the concept of psychological reversal.

Dr. Robert Blaich is a leading practitioner of Applied Kinesiologist (AK), a method of diagnosis for chiropractic problems that involves testing various muscles. AK was discovered and developed by Dr. George Goodheart, a genius chiropractor from Detroit. Dr. Blaich and his colleague, Dr. David Walther, jointly taught the hundred-hour AK course that I attended. I had discovered PR prior to taking the course. Drs. Blaich and Walther were the first health care professionals to see the value of my discovery of psychological reversal.

In his superb presentation of Applied Kinesiology, Walther (1988) states:

> Most practicing physicians can recognize psychologically reversed individuals in their practices. These are often the individuals who respond poorly to treatment: when there is some improvement in a condition, they will dwell on the negative aspects. Even when the improvement is pointed out, they will immediately change the subject back to the negative aspects.

Dr. Blaich, also an outstanding chiropractor, specializes in high-level human performance and works with a number of elite, world-class athletes. He told me he found the PR correction to be invaluable in helping these athletes to break their own and other's records.

Dr. Blaich (1988) did a most interesting research project wherein he attempted to improve the reading speed and comprehension of a group of professionals. The study used various treatment methods that might aid people who were already high achievers to improve their performance level even more. He measured and demonstrated performance by using reading and comprehension skills. He found the treatment for PR (which was by far the most rapid and simple of the various treatments used) was the *most effective* of all the therapy methods used. Some methods tested required very high professional skills in order to perform the complex procedure. He stated:

Reading #4, which provided a 45% improvement over reading #3 and a 119% improvement over reading #1, *followed the treatment for Psychological Reversal and exhibited the greatest single change in reading rate of any of the steps done. Dr. Callahan's procedure seems to have a very significant impact on human performance as evaluated here* [my emphasis]. (p.12)

The PR treatment as now used,[3] takes less than five seconds; and although other treatments were used, the PR treatment was the only TFT treatment used in this study.

PR AND CANCER

Soon after I discovered psychological reversal, I observed something interesting. My clients came to me because they had various psychological problems. During the period of 1981-83, I saw eight clients who also happened to have cancer. I noticed each of these clients showed massive PR. I thought this was an interesting finding, but did not make much of it since the number of individuals was so small.

Around this time I gave a workshop on my procedures to some interested psychologists. One of them, Dr. Lee Shulman, specialized in working with cancer patients. When I reported my finding about cancer and psychological reversal he decided to check out my finding with his larger group of cancer clients. He was seeing more

---

[3] In earlier days, I used an affirmation along with the hand tap, but I found it was completely unnecessary and misleading, and today we only tap the PR spot five times.

than 35 cancer patients at the time. Upon checking them for PR he reported that every one of these clients also showed the presence of PR. Over a longer period of time, Dr. Shulman reported he continued to find this relationship between cancer and PR.

What does this mean? I am no expert in cancer, and I know there are numerous people who show PR who do not have cancer. Nevertheless, this seemed a rather curious finding. No other diagnostic category stood out so emphatically as far as the presence of psychological reversal is concerned. After being treated for PR, a few cancer clients appeared to recover surprisingly from their cancer, but there was no way to know if any part of their recovery was helped by our treatments or not. It would make some sense if the treatments, including the treatments for PR, did help eliminate their cancer but there is insufficient evidence at this time.[4]

PROFESSOR HAROLD SAXTON BURR

A few years ago, I was able to track down a book I had been searching for by Harold Saxton Burr. Dr. Burr was a biologist at Yale University in the 1940s who did some very interesting work with a sensitive voltmeter. He demonstrated that all living things, even leaves, possessed a polarity on this meter (Burr, 1972).

---

[4] There is some support for the idea that reducing psychological stress may be a contributing factor in helping some people with cancer. It has also been shown that it can be helpful for hopeless cancer patients if they can *do* something to help themselves. We recommend every cancer patient correct their own PR numerous times throughout the day by simply tapping the PR spot on the side of the hand.

In the appendix of Burr's book is a most interesting report of the findings of Louis Langman, MD, who had been a student of Dr. Burr. Dr. Langman was a professor of gynecology at New York University and carried out a most remarkable study. He hypothesized that cancer is fundamentally an alteration of field forces in the body. To check this idea he examined cellular diagnosed cases of cancer under blind conditions (i.e., the pathologist and Dr. Langman did not know who was who). He compared these cases (in measurements of body polarity by Burr's method) to normal individuals. (The measurement of polarity was done with a sensitive voltmeter placing the electrodes on different parts of the body.) The startling results were as follows:

Those with no malignant condition

Positive polarity	74
Negative polarity	4

95% of the normal group showed the measured polarity to be positive.

Those with malignancy

Positive polarity	5
Negative polarity	118

96% of this group showed polarity to be negative.

Cancer group: 96% negative polarity
Non-cancer (normal group): 5% negative polarity

The cancer group has a striking preponderance of women showing a reversal of normal polarity. This appears to correlate with what Dr. Shulman and I found with psychological reversal. Dr. Langman then studied an additional 737 patients who had a benign gynecological condition. He found that in this group 611 showed a positive polarity and 126 were negative, (i.e., 83% positive and 17% negative). A further strong confirmation of Langman's relationship between polarity and cancer received very strong support from a fact that when cancerous tumors were removed the polarity reversed from negative to positive (Langman, in Burr 1972, p. 144).

Although these are surprisingly very high correlations, we cannot, at this point, assume any causal relationships. We do not know which comes first, cancer or PR. If I understand Langman's thinking, it would seem that the psychological or the polarity reversal may be primary in some important respect. We typically find most chronic conditions, physical or psychological, have a PR associated with them. We know most people who have a PR— we all do at times—*do not* have cancer, but nevertheless the findings are strongly suggestive. More than this cannot be said with any confidence at this time. If any published researcher with access to cancer patients would like to investigate this, I would be happy to contribute my understandings and experience to the research.

Since we find psychological problems cannot be successfully treated when there is a PR (the perturbations, P's, simply will not show), perhaps something similar exists with at least some cases of cancer. If there is a PR, then healing may be unable to take place. This may make the cancer more strongly established in the system, insulated from the ordinary healing forces.

CONTROL SYSTEM AND DIRECTION

Burr (1972) pointed out, "In the growth and development of every living system there is obviously some kind of control of the processes." (p. 58) He noted that control requires *direction* and points out one of the few things in the universe, that possesses direction is the electrical property of things. Even atypical growth (e.g., cancer) requires direction. He added that life requires energy but energy has no direction. What I call the PR and what Burr called the reversals of polarity appear to make sense from the standpoint of control forces operating within life.

SLEEP, ANESTHESIA AND PR

Robert O. Becker (1987) reported a very interesting finding: Living creatures show a polarity reversal when they sleep and when they are under anesthesia. I know from long experience with PR that a condition cannot heal if there is a PR present. Sleep and anesthesia represent two different degrees of lack of general awareness. It has been shown that some people show evidence of awareness even under anesthesia; this has been known for many years and has prompted those in the operating room to be careful of what they say in the presence of an anesthetized patient. Based on this, I would predict patients in a coma would also show a general PR but this has not been tested as far as I know.

It is interesting that the PR is an electrical and, more precisely, a polarity phenomenon. Many systems in the body take advantage of polarities in order to operate effectively. If the proper polarity is incorrect then there is a blockage of flow (just like two north poles on a magnet repel each other, instead of attraction there is repulsion). When such is the case in a healing system then we run into potentially serious problems. But remember that many of the serious problems are quite correctable with the simple correction of the PR that will then allow healing to properly begin.

Anesthesiologist Stuart Hameroff of Arizona State University, along with mathematical physicist Roger Penrose, is a major contributor to theories of understanding consciousness. Hameroff pointed out that the gases used in anesthesia are not from a common chemical category, but rather seem similar in their electric effects on the system.

I find it especially relevant in this context that recent discoveries of the process of inebriation show it is not the chemical effect of alcohol which results in drunkenness—the chemical effect *is* relevant, however, in understanding cell damage—but *rather it is the electric effect of alcohol on the brain cells* which causes drunkenness.

ALCOHOL'S ELECTRIC EFFECTS

No one has understood how intoxication takes place. It is known that ethanol does not appear to affect brain cells until the concentration is deadly and begins to destroy cells. It has been found that the body begins breaking ethanol down into fatty acid ethyl esters. These changes, it is reported, result in changes in calcium, which in turn affects the electric activity of the cells.

This landmark finding is reported in a Jan. 11, 1997 *Science News* article: "In the Dec 20, 1996, *Journal of Biological Chemistry*, by Richard Gross and Rose A. Gubatosi-Klug, of Washington University School of Medicine, Gross says: Our report is the first to show...these profound changes in the electrical functions of a [brain cell] at concentrations of alcohol which are present after people drink."

For many years I have observed it is difficult or impossible to treat someone who is inebriated. In light of these reports, not only is such a person not in very high state of awareness, but it now seems the electric effects of alcohol may render the person somewhat "asleep" and the PR may be mainly responsible for the lack of responsiveness to treatments.

Taking a cue from this, I have speculated any system in a state of psychological reversal may be considered non-functional or even "dead." When I expressed this view to Joanne, my wife and co-author, she said, "No, it is more like the system is in a coma." I believe this is a more precise expression of the condition. The important news about the PR correction is that it will revive the system to proper functioning so healing may begin.

Dr. Werner Loewenstein, Director of the Laboratory of Cell Communication at the Marine Biological Laboratory, Woods Hole, Mass. has recently published some very important findings on the communication of cells. (The maintenance of life requires enormous constant communication within the living body.) All of Loewenstein's work is interesting and I recommend this work highly to scholars in this area, but one of his findings appears to cohere with my discovery of the effects of PR. Loewenstein (1999) says:

> Let us check briefly on the performance of [these units of information reception and transmission] to see how well they measure up to that promise. First, their directionality. To get a message through a communication channel, the information flowing through it must have a direction. In the channels of our technology, the direction is given by irreversible (one-way) transmission stations. This is also true for the intercellular channels, though there may be an occasional *reversible* [my emphasis] demon too along the line. But it's the irreversible ones who bring home the bacon—they are the ones who get the message through. (pp. 194-195)

I am positing that PR may well be another meaningful name for a significant collection of "reversible demons." When the PR is corrected, with my simple treatment,[5] we then are in a position to witness the reversal being cor-

---

[5]   It is a very rare event when PR does not correct, but we have discovered the cause for this and in our advanced work we know precisely what to do about it.

rected and "the bacon being brought home."[6] Or, in other words, the healing system can now deliver the information required to heal a particular system. *Please do not allow the simplicity and ease of the PR correction mislead you to underrate its relevance and importance in all kinds of healing.*

---

[6] James Clerk Maxwell proposed the demon as an entity, which (in imagination) might overturn the most sanctified law of modern science, The Second Law of Thermodynamics. The demon was proposed as a device to help Maxwell understand the Second Law (Von Baeyer, author of *Maxwell's Demon*). Maxwell, in the 1960s, is the famous scientist who created the theory of electromagnetism and Maxwell's equation, among other things.

CHAPTER 7

THE HEALING SYSTEM

W hen we successfully eliminate the disturbing effects of a trauma or phobia, what exactly happens? The high predictability of our treatments gives us a scope into the workings of the mind and body. When we do a TFT treatment there is obviously not only a reduction on the Subjective Units of Distress (SUD) Scale, but there are bodily changes that immediately occur.

THE ROULEAU EFFECT

One of the obvious physical changes that often occurs with successful TFT is that of color coming into the face of some very pale clients. We have good reason to believe this increase in color is due to an increase of oxygen being delivered to the system. This increase takes place due to a reduction in the number of red blood cells that sometimes clump together. This clumping inhibits the ability to deliver oxygen to all the cells of the body. This is known as the Rouleau effect. Watch for it when you do TFT! I have seen the clumping of red blood cells reduce dramatically as a result of my treatment.

MEDICAL APPLICATIONS OF TFT

A growing number of physicians take the TFT training and we are finding that TFT can often be very effective in helping a number of medical conditions. Roopa Chari, MD presented a case of a tumor whose progress was being measured by prolactin level by the patient's endocrinologist. The endocrinologist told her that she would be lucky if her prolactin level went town eight to ten points in the next eight months with the treatment of parlode (bromotcriptine). Dr. Chari tested the patient for some common toxins and treated her addiction to caffeine. Soon after being treated by TFT, the patient met with her neurosurgeon and asked to have the prolactin levels checked again. The doctor tried to discourage her, claiming that it was too soon for these levels to go down, but the prolactin level had dropped 37 points in six weeks!

Dr. Gale Joslin is a VT-trained psychologist who has completed training to administer drugs as the appropriate laws are passed (he doubts now that he will ever need to prescribe drugs). He reported a case of a man with a compromised immune system. Prior to VT™ TFT treatment, lab tests were done in order to provide a base line against which to measure the treatment. His protein level was 1.2 prior to the treatment. Two days after treatment it was measured again and it was 6.5. He has kept the same diet, the same routines, etc. The only change was a new toxin treatment pioneered by Dr. Stephen Daniel and administered by Dr. Joslin. His doctor said that there must be an error and ordered another protein test. Again it came out 6.5. The normal reference range for protein is 6.0-8.3. The patient is much better!

One of our top trainees suffered from lupus, high cholesterol and enlarged heart and valve problems. As a result of applying his extensive knowledge of TFT, his tests a few months later were remarkable according to the examining physician. There was no trace of lupus. The "ANA titer" which had been positive is now negative; the doctor is baffled but stated that it is a very good prognostic sign with respect to lupus. There was no further evidence of an enlarged heart or valve problems on the second echocardiogram. The cholesterol improved from 249 to 198 in the seven months since he began treating himself.

WHY DON'T PEOPLE HEAL?

Before me is an ad for a popular New Age book *Why People Don't Heal.* Since I am writing on this very subject, I was drawn to this ad. The intriguing copy asks the central question: "Why do some people heal while others don't?" The ad says the author, a "medical intuitive," has worked with thousands of patients.

It stimulates my interest further when I read that the author has developed a "unique approach to the study of energy anatomy—the electromagnetic channels that connect mind and spirit: the 'circuitry' that is crucial to the self-healing process." Excited by the implications of those notions, I am let down terribly when I read that the reason we do not heal is because we use our illnesses (or "wounds") as a way of gaining intimacy and even personal power. This is virtually the same as theories of "secondary gain" and "resistance" offered by traditional psychology. Because successful results were not obtained with such treatments, they tend to attribute the reasons for this to deficits in the client, rather than looking for more effective treatment methods. Since I have not seen the book, I am not actually addressing the book with my critical remarks but rather the ad. The promise implicit in the wonderful phrase "energy anatomy," at least in the ad, seemed to become lost.

It is a good idea to look for and correct the psychological reversal if healing seems blocked. When a person has a disorder or condition whose natural course should result in healing, but for some strange reason does not appear to recover or the usual otherwise effective treatments do not seem to help, there may be a PR.

Psychological reversal is such a useful and potent concept that many readers encountering it for the first time may erroneously overuse it. I must point out what I mean by PR is highly specific and all problems are definitely *not* due to PR but have other types of causation. PR, in other words, is not an omnibus notion that covers everything; it is delimited, specific, and has definite features and symptoms. *There are many severe problems that have no psychological reversal accompanying them.* If PR correction does not seem to help and help is important, we recommend finding a therapist trained in TFT diagnosis or, better yet, trained in Voice Technology™. A call to our office will provide such information.

CHAPTER 8

THE APEX PROBLEM

Most men occasionally stumble over the truth, but most pick themselves up and continue on as if nothing happened.

Winston Churchill

You have learned something—that always feels, at first, as if you had lost something.

George Bernard Shaw

The apex problem is a most fascinating and predictable aspect of these treatments. The term is borrowed from Arthur Koestler (1967), who refers to the operation of mind at its peak or apex. The apex *problem* refers to the absence of same. If you are not alerted to this prevalent phenomenon in advance, you will be quite surprised and puzzled if you do very many of these treatments. We have had therapists do TFT and help their clients dramatically, but became discouraged because the clients did not give them credit for the help. When one understands the apex and is prepared for it, the effect can be minimized.

The apex problem refers to the commonly observed experience in TFT that a person who receives treatment for any particular problem will *accurately* report the expected and predicted improvement but TYPICALLY WILL NOT CREDIT THE TREATMENT for the improvement. The report of change from TFT treatment follows the predictions, but the improved individual apparently has difficulty believing the changes are due to the therapy—even though this is the express purpose of therapy! One might expect the person to be hesitant to report changes or distort or minimize the changes, but interestingly this is usually not the case. The client typically reports accurately and conforms to the laws of TFT, even though these laws are completely unknown to the client.

To qualify as an apex problem, the client must report changes. If the client does not report a change that actually takes place, this is quite a different problem than the apex. There may be a common root, such as the fact the client can hardly believe such a rapid change could take place. Rarely, a person will change but is so baffled by the phenomenon that he will not report the change. Even the skeptical and disbelieving client reports improvements regularly and accurately. How do we know they are accurate? Mainly from the behaviors that follow successful treatment.

Importance of Asking How Client Feels Now

I was supervising a trainee by telephone who was working with a difficult depressed client. I used Voice Technology™ to determine the precise treatments needed, and passed them on to the trainee, who then administered them to the client. The client was a 9 on the SUD for depression and reported no change after the treatment. A further voice analysis was done and there were no perturbations showing. The client was asked if she was sure she still felt depressed. The client said she did not feel depressed *now* but was sure she would feel depressed *tomorrow* and therefore she was reporting no change. This is why, when we ask for a SUD report during treatment, we emphasize, "How do you feel NOW, AT THIS MOMENT?"

Despite this precision in the formulation of the question, the client may easily dodge the precise question in order to express doubts. In fact, the therapist, the trainer and the client together do not know how the client will feel at some time in the future. All we have is the present, and that is why the focus is on the present in the treatment and the queries regarding treatment. A robust empirical clinical fact I've found, after treating thousands of people, is that the treatments will usually hold. Of course, in any individual case, we never know for sure until time passes.

SCIENTIFIC RELEVANCE OF IDENTIFYING
THE APEX PROBLEM

The identification of the apex phenomenon has basic scientific relevance since it *refines prediction*. Due to the apex problem, we do not predict the recipients of treatment will credit the treatment; instead, we predict they will report a dramatic change of state after the treatment. We may further predict one will *not* credit the treatment for the change but will invent other explanations in order to avoid the obvious fact of the role of treatment. Examples of other and irrelevant "explanations" for the positive treatment effect include distraction, placebo, suggestion, hypnosis, and the rewrite of history (e.g., "I never had the problem before the treatment.").

Why this avoidance of acknowledging the obvious efficacy of the treatment? It seems that in order to credit the surprisingly effective treatment, which only a small number do, it is necessary in the client's context to consider the treatment as a "miracle"! (A very small number of successfully treated individuals, who do not resort to the apex problem, may actually say, "It's a miracle!")

Miracles do not happen in contradiction of nature,
but in contradiction of what we know about nature.

Saint Augustine (1354-1430)

Since the typical recipient is not familiar with our unusual treatment, it does sometimes seem to be a miracle. A miracle is something that happens quite contrary to our expectations or what we believe we *can or ought to* expect.

The apex problem obstructs the necessity of acknowledging a miracle, that is, a result that could not have been expected or predicted given current limited conventional psychological treatments. The apex reaction avoids the necessity of thinking hard about what actually transpired and rethinking old, perhaps excessively cherished, beliefs and notions. As old-timer psychologist Edgar Doll put it: "They suffer from a hardening of the categories."

An Early Apex Problem Example with Hypnosis

I was a pioneer in clinical hypnosis. I no longer use hypnosis since TFT (totally unrelated to hypnosis) is much faster, more easily replicated by others, more generally applicable, and more powerful *as a treatment* than hypnosis. I still remain interested in hypnosis for reasons other than psychotherapy.

In the winter of 1949, I was with a group of fellow students in Ann Arbor, Michigan, studying for a final undergraduate exam in a psychology course. One of the students asked if anyone knew how to do hypnosis. I replied that I did. They wanted to see a demonstration and I asked for a volunteer. As it turned out he was an excellent and gifted hypnotic subject. Bob (who has since become a physician) was able to receive suggestions of all kinds, including positive and negative hallucinations.

I gave Bob the following posthypnotic suggestion with amnesia: When the word "psychology" was mentioned, he was to take off his shirt, but he would not remember I had told him this. What follows is an excellent illustration of the apex problem.

After Bob was taken out of the hypnotic state, he reported he felt fine. We all resumed our study for a final exam in psychology. When someone mentioned the word "psychology" all eyes surreptitiously stole to Bob, who began to appear uncomfortable. After fidgeting in his chair for a few moments he left the table and went to a window. He opened the window and let in very cold air. We told him to close the window. Bob complained the room was too hot and then proceeded to take off his shirt.

He carried out the post-hypnotic suggestion, but did not remember being told this order. Note that he introduced some creative and invented twists to the story, by opening the window and complaining about the heat. These "explanations," which he invented on the spot, allowed Bob to follow through with the act of shirt removal. He compulsively had it "make sense" by creatively and subconsciously inventing the overheating of the room.

This is what we call the "apex problem." We call it a "problem" because it effectively shuts off the person from seeing relevant evidence. It causes the person to think he "knows" the answer to something when, in fact he does not have an inkling. Even though Bob knew he had just been hypnotized, he did not mention this possibility to account for his strange behavior. He compulsively offered something which "made sense" to him. The word "compulsive" is operative here because we find therapists and others who observe TFT in action seem *compelled* to explain our results with something they believe they already understand, such as placebo, hypnosis, suggestion, or distraction. Interestingly, the successfully treated client or observer typically does not *ask* what happened, or rarely considers the rather obvious possibility that the change may have something to do with the treatment just administered in an effort to alleviate the problem. Even clients who pay money for help do not initially consider that the treatment did the job.

Neils Bohr, a major founder of quantum physics, once said that if one was not shocked when confronting quantum physics, then one did not understand it. When one quickly explains away potentially shocking information by not facing it or denying it, this suggests the apex problem may be a common way of avoiding mental shock and the necessary mental work involved. This apex solution avoids the necessary reordering of all previously held (and perhaps *unduly cherished*) information that may no longer be relevant in the light of new scientific discovery.

A Recent Example of Apex

A surgeon in his middle fifties had had a melanoma when he was a young medical student. It was successfully removed, but he developed a compulsive problem (which I consider a behavioral addiction) of checking constantly for signs of melanoma. Any slight blemish might be cancer. When he became a surgeon he would compulsively cut away any minor mark or blemish from his skin. He knew this was inappropriate but he could not help himself. He told me he had spent, over the years, some

$300,000 in intense psychoanalysis attempting to correct this problem. Although he felt he had learned a lot about himself in this lengthy enterprise, self-knowledge was not sufficient to reduce the problem. The compulsion remained, even after all the years of therapy and money spent.

He received three brief (each lasting only a few minutes) sessions of TFT, addiction treatment directed toward this compulsion. He scoffed at the strangeness and simplicity of the procedure. I did not hear from him again until three years later. He contacted me to report there had been no further trace of the compulsion since the treatment and he suddenly realized he had not performed surgery on himself since the time of the last TFT treatment. It took three years before this highly intelligent person put this together.

The apex problem is definitely not an issue of intelligence; we have had highly creative and brilliant people who resort to the apex problem rather than to acknowledge the easily demonstrated power of Thought Field Therapy.

A TFT Trainee "Forgot" He Had Depression

Even therapists trained in TFT diagnostic procedures are not immune from the apex problem. We encourage TFT-trained therapists to get help with TFT for their own problems. A recent trainee had been suffering from depression for years. Previous therapy and medications had not helped. After the first telephone therapy session, all traces of depression were completely eliminated. Two weeks later, in replying to a question about his state, the therapist said he had "forgotten" he had depression. A brief reminder was all that was needed to elicit a loud laugh and a recognition of the apex problem residing within himself! This gave an unforgettable insight into the awesome power of the apex problem, even in a therapist trained to understand it.

OTHER EXAMPLES

Lois is thinking of driving, which prompts her to experience great fear. She had previously tried drugs, psychotherapy (four different therapies), and meditation, but she still is terrified at the mere thought of driving. She reported that for the last ten years, she has been unable to think about driving without breaking down. Lois usually goes to a 10 now, merely *thinking about* driving.

We gave her a TFT treatment. Suddenly, she said, "Oh, I can't think about it right now." The therapist said, "Well, just take a few moments to think about it and see if you can get yourself as upset as you did before the treatment."

"No," she reported, "I can't get upset because you distracted me with all those things you had me do." The therapist patiently explained that at this moment she was not doing those things. Lois then explained there have been times in the past when she would not get upset about driving. This is directly contradictory with what she had reported *before* the treatment (i.e., that she could never even think about the issue without getting extremely upset). She then threw in another common comment: "But of course I'm not upset right now because I'm just sitting here talking to you." The therapist tried again, "Yes, but remember you were just sitting here talking to me a few minutes ago, when you were at a 10 on the 10-point scale." No strategy could get Lois to consider the therapy, whose *express purpose* was to eliminate the problem, played any role in the rather wonderful event.

Another apex example happened on a radio show in Missouri, where I was a guest via telephone. The host had received information about my work and had asked his teenage daughter to appear on the show. She apparently had some problem that did not respond to conventional therapy and he wanted to see if I could help her.

After talking to me a few minutes, it was clear he was quite skeptical, which is perfectly understandable. Initial skepticism is not in any way an aspect of the apex problem, but is a quite normal reaction to startling claims. He asked me if I would demonstrate the treatment on his daughter. I explained it was not necessary for her to talk about the problem but to merely think about it while I checked her voice (with our proprietary diagnostic Voice Technology™).

She reported a 10 just thinking about this problem and that this was typical since the problem began two years earlier. After treatment she was thrilled (no apex problem). She said her problem did not bother her at all, and asked if this result was likely to last. I said it probably would last, but of course, we don't know for sure until time passes.

On the other hand, her father seemed to become somewhat angry and upset by the success. He proclaimed his disbelief of the treatment and then, unfortunately, accused his daughter of lying about her improvement. It seemed he would prefer to believe his daughter had lied than to accept the possibility that the treatment had worked!

Another memorable apex event was when I was asked to appear on a show in Minneapolis, near the University of Minnesota. I was warned that if I accepted the challenge of treating volunteers with phobias on this show, I would also have to face the chief of psychiatry from the university's medical school. He had read my book *The Five Minute Phobia Cure* and was very critical of my claims. I said I welcomed his presence.

I traveled to Minnesota. The psychiatrist had some nice things to say about my book until, he said, it came to the treatment part. He explained it is impossible to cure phobias with *any* treatment, let alone the peculiar treatments I had presented in my book. "These treatments are beyond the pale," he explained.

He characterized each of the three volunteer phobics as "severe," as they indeed were. One lady had such a severe fear of heights she had to live in a basement because she could not live on a first floor. She was in obvious agony as she bravely went up two steps of a ladder that was on the set prior to the treatment. In a few minutes, the startled and thrilled volunteer appeared to be completely over her severe phobia. She did not show an apex problem, but commented after the treatment, "That is really something that this doctor did. I don't know what it was but it sure worked!"

The other two volunteers, a very severe cat phobic and a spider phobic were also dramatically helped. The chief of psychiatry announced that these cures were a result of what he called "show biz." He did not say *before* I did the treatment that show biz—whatever that is—would cure a phobia. In fact he said that *nothing* could cure a phobia. This was a *rapid apex solution* to his problem— the conviction that no therapy, let alone the strange-appearing TFT therapy, could cure phobias.

Perhaps it is now clear why the person who does our treatments must be familiar with the apex problem. Note that the apex problem does not typically interfere with accurate reporting of positive change due to the therapy. It applies to the *interpretation* or "explanation" of *why* there was change. Also keep in mind that identification of the apex problem not only prepares us for some surprising and shocking reactions to TFT, but also *refines our predictions* as mentioned earlier and therefore has basic scientific value.

SPLIT BRAIN

Some people who suffer from severe epileptic seizures receive a treatment for this condition consisting of cutting the commisure that connects the two separate hemispheres of the brain. These people present an interesting problem in that they appear to have two separate minds. Dr. Michael Gazzaniga (1985) has studied these people carefully and notes they show something quite similar to what we call the apex problem. Examples of the same phenomenon are shown with split-brain subjects and are cited by Dr. Gazzaniga who says "the normal human is compelled to interpret real behaviors and to construct a theory as to why they have occurred." (p. 74)

Dr. Gazzaniga considers this confabulation due to what he calls the "left-brain interpreter." In his split-brain experiments, he discovered that the language aspect of the left brain will invent and create "explanations" for phenomena that are introduced to the non-verbal right brain and not known to the left. However, the left brain, observing the behavior, will compulsively "explain" what is taking place even though there is no factual basis for the "explanation." It is pure irrelevant invention. They never seem to wonder about the possible role of their surgery, in the same manner as the successfully treated person ignores the role of the therapy, along with its implied prediction. Similarly, Bob, the hypnotized subject mentioned earlier ignored the fact he had been hypnotized.

It seems evident in TFT treatment that the "brain" is confronted with a phenomenon it cannot comprehend—immediate successful treatment—and the "left brain" in Gazzaniga's terms, begins inventing irrelevant "explanations." This happens even though in the TFT treatment the commisure connecting the brain's hemispheres is intact and there is no hypnosis or induced amnesia. This phenomenon probably occurs in most of us at times and its commonplace nature will become obvious to anyone using these treatments. If the individual were functioning at or near the apex of the mind (which is rare for all of us), the explanations compulsively offered in an apex problem would not be acceptable. The compulsion for a familiar and effortless "explanation" appears to override critical thinking in the attempt to grasp something entirely new and unfamiliar.

The speed and stunning effectiveness of TFT seems to generate the apex problem. Nothing the subject has known before could account for the result. Therefore (and you will especially find this among psychotherapists), they will compulsively *tell you, not ask you* why the change took place. Favorites among the compulsive explanations are placebo effect, hypnosis, or distraction. That the therapist himself has never witnessed similar demonstrations of the power of placebo, hypnosis, or distraction, appears to carry little weight.

We have found that explanations about the apex problem before treatment appear to have little effect upon reducing its occurrence, although some written material and even tape recordings of the treatment session may be used to advantage. As TFT and its results become more generally known and accepted, we expect the apex problem to evaporate.

Apex Problem among Therapists

In the last few years I have presented at a number of professional meetings and often I'll give live demonstrations with volunteers from the attendees. I present information about TFT, including my rather startling claims of high success. Then, a volunteer from the audience, usually a professional therapist, presents a problem that has not responded to previous therapy attempts. It is extremely rare to have a failure in these demonstrations.

Incident: A therapist, with no formal training in TFT but who knows some TFT algorithms, is talking to a group of about ten psychologist-therapists in San Francisco following a major earthquake in the area. The discussion naturally goes to the psychological effects of the quake and about a third of the group report they still suffer some trauma effects. The therapist immediately gives them a demonstration and each therapist was completely symptom-free. They are, of course, surprised by this result. They have never heard of TFT, but are given my name and told of my work. I never heard from any of them.

Why is this surprising? Well, they were not taught how to do the algorithm. It must have seemed like a confusing bit of hocus-pocus to them. But, they all had patients who suffered from the trauma of the earthquake. Since they were helped almost magically and immediately, doesn't it seem reasonable at least one of them might want to hear more about the procedure in order to help his own clients? Immediately, most people assume the therapists were money-motivated and would not want their clients to get off so easily. This might be a consideration for some, but certainly not for all. I believe their lack of interest is more often due to the apex problem. They are not able to actually perceive what the therapy accomplished due to mental manipulations that separate them from the experience.

It took me a number of years before I saw the connection of the apex problem in reaction to my treatments and the hypnosis episode of almost 50 years earlier. The apex problem was the last thing I would have expected from the numerous people who, unresponsive to conventional therapies, are almost instantly cured of their problem with TFT. Who would ever imagine these people would *deny* the treatment that was consciously and explicitly done to help them had any bearing upon their success?

Once in a great while a successfully treated client gets hostile after his or her problem is gone, almost as if he or she thinks you played a dirty joke. An accomplished magician once told me that he appreciated my enthusiasm and appreciation of his skilled magicianship. He added something surprising which I could later relate to: Sometimes when he did a wonderful magic trick he would encounter hostility from an observer. He asked me for my psychological opinion on this. I said I did not know why this was, but perhaps these people suffered from some kind of inferiority feelings. Possibly they thought they *ought* to know how the trick was done and felt somewhat stupid for feeling fooled. Of course most people's appreciation of good magic is that they enjoy the wonderment and surprise of seemingly impossible tricks being done. When knowledge of TFT becomes more widespread, we expect the apex problem to simply fade away. Most people will, as most TFT therapists do, expect a client to start getting dramatically better with the first treatment.

CHAPTER 9

THE SUD SCALE:
HOW WE MEASURE
SUCCESS WITH TFT

SUBJECTIVE UNITS OF DISTRESS (SUD)

The use of the Subjective Units of Distress Scale (SUD) is a common 10- or 11-point scale, attributed to Dr. Joseph Wolpe,[1] denoting how one feels. The SUD is indispensable in evaluating clinically significant psychotherapy because this is a measure that has broad applicability. For example, some years ago I mea-

---

[1] As a graduate director of an Office of Naval Research project while at Syracuse University, I was privileged to work with Eric Gardner, dean of the Graduate School, and George G. Thompson, psychology professor, and my dissertation advisor. These two eminent scholars had devised a human rating 10-point scale, which was far more sophisticated than the SUD in that it was designed to be used in advanced statistics and research and had features which made this possible.

sured blood pressure on all my clients before and after treatment. The vast majority of those whose blood pressure was above normal experienced an immediate, dramatic drop in their blood pressure into the low-normal range.

One particularly severely anxious client went off the blood pressure scale—the scale did not go high enough—when thinking of her fear. The automatic printout machine did not register high enough. Immediately after the brief TFT treatment, she showed a low-normal reading. However, a considerable number of clients began with a low-normal reading prior to therapy and thus showed no change in blood pressure due to treatment—there was nowhere for the blood pressure to go.

As an additional problem with using blood pressure as a measure of treatment success, a small percentage of those whose blood pressure dramatically declined after therapy still were as anxious after the therapy as before, though this was before I advanced the treatments to the technical level they are today. This situation struck me as similar to the old line, "The operation was a success but the patient died." As Professor Magda Arnold (1960) of Loyola pointed out decades ago, there is no physiological measure that can accurately reflect or convey the emotions a person experiences. This is similar to the difficulty in measuring physical pain; there is absolutely no valid substitute for the client's report. These facts are related to a major reason lie detection is not accepted in courts of law and why insurance investigators for possible fraud are required to provide direct evidence showing the claimant doing things he states he cannot do. Psychotherapists, as indicated by the very name, are involved in treating the subjective upsetting feelings or emotions of their clients. There is not now, and I doubt there ever can be, a direct objective substitute for the client's report.[2] Early in my career I treated a few people who were referred because they had pain. Some experts told them it was in their head. At first I treated them in the usual ways and this did not help their pain. Finally, I referred them to other specialists and, in two out of the three cases, a serious source of pain was discovered. One pain case, the internist said, would have died in another week. One lung had collapsed, which was not observed by two different physicians, and the good lung would have been out of order soon.

"How Are You Today?"

This common human query is a universal greeting. Typically, answers are vague, such as "Fine." In therapy, when we ask how someone is in a treatment situation, we ask him or her to assign numbers—usually from 1 to 10. Ten is the worst one can be and 1 is "fine" or "no trace of a problem." In my psychological graduate education, it was apparent to me there was a kind of taboo against simply asking clients how they are. Elaborate scales and inventories have been developed and are often used in-

---

[2] Perhaps the best instrument with promise is the Heart Rate Variability, which, among other things, shows the balance of the autonomic nervous system. But as helpful as this instrument is—and it is the best of those which I am aware—it is still no substitute for the report of the person as to how he or she feels.

stead of asking the simple, direct question. Often the inventories are just another method, but seemingly more elaborate, of asking clients to tell us how they are. I prefer the SUD in most cases.

In treating infants, animals, or very young children one cannot obtain a SUD report. They need to be treated in a real situation because they cannot be directed to "think of" the situation (i.e., tune the thought field). In such cases, upsetting exposure should be titrated to the lowest level possible in order to minimize needless suffering. Upset is not a part of TFT treatment; we try to avoid it or keep it to an absolute minimum whenever possible.

WHY USE NUMBERS?

If you remember the Woody Allen movie comedy *Annie Hall,* there was a scene where the protagonists were shown on a split screen with their respective therapists, who were asking about their sex lives. Annie replied it was just terrible: "We have sex all the time! That's all we ever do!" "How frequently?" asked the quantitatively minded therapist. *"Twice a week,"* replied Annie. Woody's therapist asked the same question and Woody replied, "We hardly ever have sex!" "How infrequently?" asked the therapist. Woody replied, *"Twice a week."* This sort of discrepancy in description illustrates why the therapist would rather have a scalar report since non-numerical adjectives may have such a wide range of different meanings.

When I used conventional therapies in treating phobias, I would teach my clients how to relax, challenge their beliefs about the issue they were unreasonably afraid of, hypnotize them (giving them good suggestions), and gradually increase the amount of exposure to the frightening situation over weeks and months.

The client would gradually improve his or her *actions*. They would go closer to the snake, drive over the bridge, look out the window in a high building, haltingly touch the bug or snake, or climb up the ladder. However, when I asked them how they felt when doing these actions, they would report they felt terrible—the SUD was still high. I gradually realized the treatment was not eliminating the fear; it was just kind of coercing the client to do things they did not want to do. This torture treatment taught them that they could take more suffering than they thought they could. TFT does much more than this. TFT typically eliminates all traces of the problem at the deepest level— the perturbation is collapsed and when treatment is complete all suffering is gone.

DEMAND CHARACTERISTIC OF SUD

The "demand characteristic" of SUD refers to a concern among some critical therapists that when you ask people how they are, they may tell you what you want to hear rather than what actually *is*. Of course, in the seemingly very peculiar TFT procedures, *the demand characteristics are quite the opposite of this tendency.* The pressure is not to report accurately, but despite this pressure, most do report accurately.

The powerful internal pressure on the person successfully treated with TFT is clearly to *not* respond with pleasing the therapist, but surprisingly (in this context) the client reports accurately that the problem is gone *despite* this *counter-demand characteristic.* This counter-demand characteristic is made very clear in the apex problem.

Do people ever give a false improvement report in TFT when there has been no improvement at all? Yes, but this is extremely rare. As mentioned earlier, we have a number of internal checks in TFT on the accuracy of the client's report. One of these checks is that a false report is usually of 1 point of SUD improvement. Although one point of improvement may be accurate in certain rare cases where there is a very complex problem, it is automatically suspect in TFT. Rarely do "positive thinkers" report that the SUD goes from a 10 to a 1; they know better. They may want to please you but they don't want to appear crazy. It is fascinating that people typically report accurately how they feel even when dramatic, immediate and radical improvements are taking place.

CHAPTER 10

CURE AND TIME

In addressing the non-hard fields of science, the famous physicist Richard Feynman stated, "You see, we in this field [physics] have a tremendous advantage over people in some other fields because we experiment to check our ideas." (Davies and Brown, p. 202)

A more concise expression of how TFT was developed is not possible. TFT has experimental advantage over all other treatments. In fact, I have often observed that the great advantage I have had in developing both my causal diagnosis and my treatments is that I was guided *totally* by the immediate results of the therapy experiments I carried out. The fact that I did my best to ignore all my prejudices and expectations based upon my many years of clinical experience and previous misunderstandings gave me the powerful edge, which made the development of TFT possible.

Every single aspect of TFT was developed by the clinical experiments I carried out over a period of two decades. Many modifications were dropped because they had little or no impact on the results as measured by the client report, which was my bottom line. Since the results of my treatments are immediate, an unprecedented rapid feedback took place that immediately informed me of the impact of any particular treatment I was investigating.

When TFT is done correctly, no other form of help can come close to our success rate. This rate has been climbing through the years, thanks to the continuing new discoveries I have made. Each of these discoveries through the last two decades contributes to the growing success rate. In the last year and a half, for example, I have made three new discoveries in Voice Technology™ (VT) which have increased our already astonishingly high success rates to even higher levels. Some of the VT trainees were able to participate in the testing of these recent discoveries. The high success rate has permitted me to reasonably introduce the concept of "cure" to the field of mental health. Cure was not listed in the dictionaries of psychiatry and psychology I consulted.

In 1993 Adler wrote an article for the *American Psychological Association Monitor*, quoting a number of experts from the Science Directorate who proclaimed cure was impossible! Well, to again quote one of my favorite scientists, Feynman: "Science is belief in the ignorance of experts." Feynman is speaking here not of humdrum everyday stuff that comes under the name of science, but was referring to creative science, the startling new discoveries which the hum drum every day world of the conventional science technician knows nothing about.

Orville Wright offered a similar notion to Feynman's when he said, "If we all worked on the assumption that what is accepted as true is really true, there would be little hope for advance."

Interestingly, even after he and his brother successfully were flying for several years, the experts were still contending that man would never fly.

DEFINITION OF CURE

Cure is a term that is rarely, if ever, mentioned in psychology. I never used the term myself until my discovery of the *Five Minute Phobia Cure* over a decade and a half ago. Dr. Joseph Wolpe, a pioneer in behavior therapy used "cure" in the subtitle of a book he co-authored with his son (1988), though I could not find the word in the index or anywhere in the book.

My usage of "cure" was necessitated by the fact that all traces of a phobia, as well as sequelae, such as nightmares, were gone after the TFT treatment. The usual definitions of cure contain several different meanings:

1. Recovery or relief from disease; 2. a course or period of treatment; 3. to restore to health; 4. something that corrects, heals or permanently alleviates a harmful or troublesome situation; 5. to free from something objectionable or harmful; 6. to rectify an unhealthy or undesirable condition; 7. successful remedial treatment; 8. to relieve or rid of something

troublesome or detrimental, as an illness, a bad habit, etc.

A cure for a psychological problem is herein defined as the complete elimination of all subjective units of distress (SUD) as well as all other symptoms associated with the problem. In TFT diagnosis, the cure state is perfectly correlated with the complete absence of perturbations as revealed in causal diagnosis.

Cure can mean to relieve or reduce a problem, although I use the term "help" in order to distinguish this lesser effect from the more complete implication of the term cure. Help means to relieve; to change for the better; a source of aid; and should be used when a treatment or series of treatments produce improvements which, though quite definite, are not quite complete.

I studiously avoided the term cure for decades, but was forced to change by the evidence of my treatments. For example, most simple phobias treated with TFT showed no trace of the phobia after the brief treatment. Following the discovery, there have been thousands of acid tests of the robustness and endurance of the treatment. Clearly, here was indeed a cure in the fullest sense of the word. The fact that the term had hardly if ever been used in psychology was irrelevant to the startling new and easily repeated facts revealed by the TFT treatments.

How Cures are Undone

Our definition of cure puts a focus on the very important fact of eliminating all symptoms of a problem. After the cure has been established, it then *and only then*, becomes possible to observe the undoing of a cure.[1] The next relevant stage in complete treatment is to evaluate the endurance of the cure over time—in TFT we call this stage of treatment "tracking." If the problem should return—a rare event—we then re-treat it in minutes but, more importantly, we find the cause of the return so it can be prevented in the future.

Margie Profet (1991) offers a new view of allergies, which makes good sense from an evolutionary standpoint. She maintains allergies are due to toxins, i.e., poisons, and that the typical allergic response is defensive and an attempt to minimize or rid oneself of the toxin. Many experts for years have maintained most allergies are a result of the immune system gone haywire since the person is reacting badly to something that is not harmful. Interestingly, this change in view parallels my own change in the phobia domain. Earlier I drew a comparison (Callahan, 1985) between an allergy (reaction to a "harmless substance") with a phobia (fear reaction to a harmless situation or object). I thought a phobia was analogous to an allergy; the difference is that it was the fear system instead of the immune system that was haywire. I later changed my view on this matter. I now believe all phobias are inherited and come from the distant past and the needed fear of a once-harmful action or thing.

---

[1] Conventional therapies are unable to view the *return* of a problem since they are unable to quickly and completely eliminate it (Adler, 1993). It is a major step forward to be able to discuss the return of a problem.

The major point of Profet's brilliant work is food toxins (or sensitivities) are actually due to poisons. Even though some people, perhaps most, can handle them with ease—some people cannot. This is a very important fact for those who believe they can cure allergies or food sensitivities. This premise should be approached with caution. Even though the person may no longer react immediately, it should not be forgotten that the real toxin might possibly cause harm in the future.

Williams and Nesse (1991) point out that plants' and vegetables' main defense against predators is to make a toxin that will discourage predation. Some of the toxic-like chemicals become neutralized when it is an advantage for the plant to have the fruit eaten. For example, some nuts are terribly poisonous until ripe, and even apples taste very sour until they ripen. This process ensures maximum spread of seeds while protecting the unripe seeds.

C.W. Smith said "When biological systems are under good control (homeostasis) the effects (of toxins) do not get larger as stress is raised, they become more complicated."[2] Contained within this simple statement is an explanation of the role of toxins in psychological problems and, specifically, why some people show complex problems.

A possible description of how toxins might create disorder was described in 1995 by Jerry Yin: "The really startling thing here is that manipulating just one molecule can perturb such complicated behavior.... There are a million ways you can muck something up...[but] if you

---

[2] Alas, I am unable to find the reference.

can improve a process, you're probably looking at something that's crucial." (p. 253) I believe a similar type of process is also relevant for our treatments.

INCIDENT

You treat a severe trauma. No symptoms remain. It looks like a complete cure. However, a few minutes after the client leaves your office, you hear a knock on the door. The client says, "A terrible thing happened—when I approached my car, the problem came back!" This is not a commonplace occurrence in TFT; it is rare with trauma treatment, but it can happen. Of course, there can be no such thing as the *return* of a problem unless it had first been gone.

What might have caused this unusual situation where all symptoms of a problem are gone and then they suddenly reappear? The details of understanding what is going on require diagnostic training, but a general understanding is possible without that specialized knowledge.

Years ago I was invited on the Tom Snyder television show to demonstrate my therapy. Tom had a very severe fear of heights and the simple phobia treatment did not work. I corrected the PR and this allowed the treatment to work. After the brief treatment (he only allowed me two minutes before the show would be over!) all traces of fear were gone. He climbed the ladder, which he could not do earlier. He was very pleased. Three years later, a colleague appeared on Tom's show and asked him about the ladder. Tom said that it worked for that day but the next day the problem returned. I had asked him to call me if his fear returned, but he didn't.

I attended a meeting where an author I knew was going to lecture on a book that had just been published. I could see she was a nervous wreck while waiting for her talk to begin. I saw her get up to go to the restroom and I went over to her. I told her I had a new discovery and asked if she would like to experience it. I explained that we might be able to quickly help her with her obvious fear. She did not seem interested but complained that she deeply regretted agreeing to give this talk. She said she'd rather "be boiled alive in oil."

I treated her and asked how she felt; she appeared much more relaxed. She went to the restroom and returned to her place at the head of the table. I was pleased to see she looked even more relaxed. When it came time to speak she said that she really enjoyed being at the meeting and she was looking forward to giving more talks because it was such an enjoyable thing to do.

Quite a switch! I expected her to say, "And thank you, Dr. Callahan, for your marvelous help." After the meeting, I went up to her and commented, "That treatment really helped, didn't it!" She said, "What treatment? You didn't do anything!" (This is yet another example of what we call the apex problem—see Chapter 8). In any case, recalling what I said after her talk, she called me two weeks later because she had a scheduled talk and was a nervous wreck. I treated her again and the same thing happened.

Later, I realized most of the people I treated stayed treated but there was one common feature shared by the author with the fear of public speaking and Tom Snyder with the fear of heights. They smoked cigarettes. I didn't know it then, but I now know that this was exactly what undid the powerful work of the treatment.

Cigarettes are a common toxin for most people but we also occasionally find there are a small number of smokers whose treatment is *not* undone by smoking a cigarette. Toxins are a very important and neglected aspect in psychotherapy, and we find that knowledge about toxins is vital to successful psychotherapeutic work. (See the 1996 article by Martha Miller; the book put out by the American Psychological Association on toxins [Travis, et al, 1989]; and the work of Doris Rapp, MD [1991], pediatric allergist.)

The most common reason for the return of a problem is not, as many therapists assume, due to psychological incidents but is rather almost always due a toxin in the form of a particular food sensitivity. Exposure to heavy doses of chemical toxins may also cause a problem to return. When the reason(s) for the return of a problem is discovered and another successful treatment is administered, it will have a good chance of being sustained over time as long as the food toxin is avoided for at least two months.

This period of abstinence gives the treated system a chance to heal with no toxic interference. I am often asked, "Do I have to stay away from the toxin forever?" We find two months free of the damaging toxin is usually adequate to ensure the problem does not return. However, I tell all my clients they would do well to be cautious about the toxin in the future for even though the treated system is now healed and the problem will not likely return, there are other consequences regarding toxins (see Rapp, 1991).

The undoing of a cure has naturally received little or no attention in psychotherapy due to the rare nature of cure itself. If one cannot cure a problem then it is meaningless to discuss the undoing of a cure. The focus on undoing a cure, a rare but definite event, has allowed us to increase our general effectiveness by identifying and avoiding exogenous causes of the major factors, which interfere with successful treatment.

Interestingly, we see the undoing of a cure, which represents a higher developmental state to be similar in principle to what in biology is called an *atavism*. An atavism is a term used in biology that refers to a throwback to an earlier ancestral form. An example is a human born with a tail or extra nipples. *Atavisms can be created in the laboratory by exposing an organism to toxins.* We believe something quite similar takes place when the previously cured state of a psychological problem is overturned. I think of a problem whose cure has been undone as a psychological atavism. The difference is that we can again treat the problem, avoid the toxin this time, and then the cure remains.

The concepts in this chapter are extremely important for a TFT therapist. Other therapies do not get cures with the regularity found in TFT and are, therefore, not in a position to observe the undoing of a cure. The knowledge of the role of toxins allows us to help people who couldn't be helped before and increases the endurance of our cures. When the undoing of a previous cure takes place, we investigate the important and neglected issue of exogenous causes, which can regenerate a problem. If one could *not* eliminate all symptoms of a problem, the recurrence and the power of tracking or searching for the causes for the recurrence would not be apparent. Rapid, effective treatments, therefore, serve as a new scope into the workings of the mind and open new vistas of great potential understanding in clinical psychology.

Investigating the role of toxins in undoing a cure has been a fruitful new way of examining our data in TFT. It has led to generating continuing improvements in the power and enhancing the understanding of the treatments. This same model could well offer similar help in fields other than psychotherapy.

For example, in this light, we might name something a cure for cancer if, after a treatment process, there remains no trace whatsoever, in careful biopsies and cell analyses of cancer cells. It seems reasonable to call the treatment that removed all traces of cancer a cure, even though the time span is only minutes rather than years. This leaves open the *important but quite separate notion* associated with the concept of cure: how long will the cure endure?

This step recognizes the fundamental fact that *any cure must begin at some point in time* and the endurance of the cure over time must be seen as an important but quite separate issue. In other words, *if a cure does not begin at some point in time, it cannot be a cure.*

A conservative colleague told me a cure should last forever. However, that definition is useless. Even if we modified the notion to mean for a lifetime, we would have to wait until our clients die before the word "cure" can be used. Even then, we never know for a certainty whether the cure might have been undone if the client had lived another minute! I feel that my proposal for the usage of cure is highly practical and meaningful.

If we have a person who gets quite upset when *merely thinking* of a situation and then, after the treatment, *under the same circumstances* (i.e., merely thinking about the problem) the person is unable to generate even the slightest upset, then I propose that we are entitled to call this a cure. How long it lasts is an entirely separate, though relevant, issue.

There are at least two pertinent issues that immediately follow after all traces of a problem and its sequelae are removed: 1) the endurance of this cure over time; 2) the testing or "proving" of the cure under various stringent circumstances or exposures, especially when treating phobias, panic, or anxiety disorders.

Calling this achievement a cure has the advantage of bestowing significance upon a treatment that can quickly eliminate all traces of a symptom. It boldly claims a vital result of treatment and marks the beginning of time when the symptoms are gone. This allows us to be on the lookout for, and to undertake an investigation into the possible specific factors that can undo a cure. These procedures have been responsible for a dramatic increase in our success rate. No longer does a client need to be discouraged if a problem returns because I now know, *in principle*, what is the cause.

If a person is pronounced free of cancer today at 3:00 PM, by testing all relevant involved tissues, and there is no discernible trace of cancerous cells, I propose the term cure be used. However, if the next day cancerous cells recur, instead of merely despairing that the treatment did not last and perhaps dismissing the important—though briefly enduring—cure, an intense investigation could be carried out to discern *why* the cure was undone. Among other things, this process recognizes the important fact that nothing can *last* or endure unless it first *is*. *It is not a weakness in a cure if a cured problem returns.*

How Long Will it Last?

Many skeptical observers will disparagingly ask after a cure, "Yes, but how long will it last?" The question is fundamental, of course, but needs to be seen objectively and not as a criticism of a treatment that can do some-thing previous treatments could not do (i.e., the complete elimination of all symptoms). Although I treated patients for over three decades prior to my discoveries, I never once heard the question, "How long will it last?" Since the discovery of TFT, I have heard this question thousands of times. Whether intended or not, it is a supreme compli-ment to ask this question. It implicitly acknowledges some-thing of significance happened in order to wonder about the duration. In TFT we carefully track our successfully treated clients and, should the problem return, which is empirically a rare event, we then set out to find an exogenous cause for this event.

In TFT it is empirically known, from wide clinical experience spanning two decades, the treatment effect usually lasts. Further, it is known this endurance will usually persist even in the face of harsh acid tests carried out in reality. For example, one anxiety client could not drive on highways because he was afraid of getting trapped in traffic. He had *two* acid tests: the first was a great fire which caused a huge traffic jam that lasted for hours, and the second, which took place two years later, was the San Francisco earthquake which created an even longer delay in traffic. These were instances of his worst nightmares come true and he showed no trace of anxiety during these two experiences after his successful treatment. He may be heard on the audiotape "Telephone Therapy," which is available from our office. Regardless of endurance, however, any cure must begin at some point in time and the present discussion highlights this important and neglected consideration.

CHAPTER 11

PLACEBO EFFECT

The magnitude and frequency of the placebo effect is unfounded and grossly overrated, if not entirely false.

G. Kienle and H. Kiene

When they first encounter the rather surprising power of TFT, a number of people will usually, without critical thought, say the result must be placebo effect. To fully understand this issue, it is first necessary to look at how "placebo" is defined. Since this word has recently been used to describe a wide variety of phenomenon, its original meaning often gets distorted.

Definitions of placebo:

Definition from the Psychiatric Glossary (APA, 1980): "The production or enhancement of psychological or physical effects using pharmacologically inactive substances administered under circumstances in which suggestion leads the subject to believe a particular effect will occur." (p. 107)

From Dictionary of Psychology (1985): "a preparation, often in pill form, used as a control in experiments requiring the administration of drugs. The placebo, which is made of sugar, acts as a control on possible suggestive effects from the knowledge that one is getting a drug." (p. 342)

Campbell (1994) quotes Wolf, who gives a broader definition of placebo: "any effect attributable to a pill, potion, or procedure, but not to its pharmacodynamic or specific properties." (p. 230)

Is TFT Placebo?

TFT may be placebo effect by the definition cited by Campbell above, which is paraphrased to fit TFT: "A procedure whose effect is not due to pharmacodynamic qualities." By this definition anything that is not an active drug is placebo and any form of effective psychotherapy would be placebo effect.

Placebo has been a mystery for years. It is assumed to be the cause of cures, including even of cancer, which is presumably due to some kind of mysterious and unknown healing power within. The cure rate by placebo is certainly not high, but is in the very low range. Cure of hopeless cancer by placebo (or unknown reason) takes place, but is very rare. It is believed to be due to a faith or confidence in a procedure or a strong belief within the person that his condition will heal. Indeed, Seligman (1994) states all effective treatments require belief or confidence in order to work. There is a certain irony when TFT is examined against this background. When people first encounter TFT there is great skepticism; it is not a treatment that engenders confidence; quite the contrary.

For those who still maintain the placebo effect is real, they must take into account that the usual precondition for placebo success is a deep belief in the procedure, pill, or whatever is being used as treatment and/or the person administering the treatment. A strong belief on the part of the client, the doctor, or preferably both is required.

Militant Skeptic Treats Militant Skeptic

Soon after my very early discoveries in TFT, I gave a workshop for a group of professionals. Naturally, there were militant skeptics in this group. I chose a militant skeptic to treat (using an algorithm) another militant skeptic with an intense trauma problem. As predicted, the trauma went from a SUD of 10 to a 1 despite the skepticism of both the therapist and the client. This did not, however, convert the skeptics to believers but it certainly gave them both pause. If belief in TFT were a requirement for success, TFT would never have gotten off the ground because it goes against all the conventional common beliefs of what is required in psychotherapy.

Further, TFT, which is so fast, powerful and unexpected in its results, generates the surprising apex problem. This is when a person is treated successfully, even though the therapy implies improvement and indeed even *predicts* improvement or cure, the successfully treated person will often deny the therapy was responsible. So we have an ironical negative placebo effect that results in a cured client who denies the treatment was responsible!

In my years of therapy prior to TFT, I would use anything that could possibly help a client with a problem, including suggestion, placebo and hypnosis. I found these procedures might offer a little help once in a while, but I never saw a cure and the degree of success of placebo was extremely small. To hear the claim of placebo effect by a therapist one would get the impression placebo cures for psychological problems are commonplace; in fact *placebo cures are so rare I have never seen it demonstrated in my long career.* I once carried out an informal survey of three additional therapists of my vintage, and they, too, reported never seeing a placebo cure a palpable problem.

My clinical observations were recently supported by the work of Kienle and Kiene (1996) of The Institute for Applied Epistemology and Medical Methodology of Freiburg, Germany. They did an analysis of over 800 studies that had claimed placebo success rates of 30 to 100%. They concluded: "The truth is that the placebo effect is counterfeited by a variety of factors, including the natural history of the disease, regression to the mean, concomitant treatments, obliging reports, experimental subordination, severe methodological defects in the studies, misquotations, etc.; even on occasion, by the fact that the supposed placebo is actually not a placebo, but has to be acknowledged as having a specific action on the condition for which it was being given. A further reason for misjudgment is the lack of clarity of the placebo concept itself..." (p. 39)

They added, "The authors conclude that the literature relating to *the magnitude and frequency of the placebo effect is unfounded and grossly overrated, if not entirely false* [my emphasis]." (p. 39)

I highly recommend anyone concerned with research and the placebo effect carefully read the article by Kienle and Kiene.

CHAPTER 12

THE PERTURBATION (P): THE FUNDAMENTAL CAUSE OF EMOTIONAL SUFFERING

[W]e have introduced a concept that is new in the context of physics—a concept that we shall call active information. The basic idea of active information is that a form having very little energy enters into and directs a much greater energy. The activity of the latter is in this way given a form similar to that of the smaller energy.

D. Bohm and B.J. Hiley

We cannot make any formal statement about a natural object (or physical system) without "getting in touch" with it. This "touch" is a real physical interaction...even if we only look at it.

Erwin Schroedinger
Founder of the basic mathematical equation in quantum physics

The laws of quantum mechanics cannot be formulated...without recourse to the concept of consciousness.

E. Wigner
Quantum physicist

John thinks about a trauma that happened 10 years ago. Merely thinking of this event results in John becoming very upset. Even though the trauma occurred a decade earlier, whenever John thinks about it, he *always* gets very upset. The simple TFT algorithm or recipe for trauma is given. When the treatment is ended, minutes later, the thought has lost the capacity to trigger the upset. This was a terrible event, but no matter how hard John tries he can no longer get upset. What happened?

To understand precisely what took place one must grasp the notion of what I call a *perturbation* (P). My view is that effective therapy—any effective therapy—collapses the perturbation(s) in the thought field. When the P or P's are collapsed, there can be no emotional upset.

There is obviously an entity residing in or carried by the thought field, that generates and controls upset. The evidence for this, in the above example, is that when the trauma is thought about, John, who was not at all upset before thinking of the trauma, gets very upset. A few minutes later, after the effective treatment, John thinks about the same trauma and not only does not get upset but, when challenged, is *unable* to get upset. It seems clear that since the same thought can be tuned, one time with upset, and the next with no upset, that something is different in the thought field after successful therapy.

This fact has been known for about 20 years, but I did not know what to call the entity in the thought field that generated the disturbance until about five years ago. When naming something new, one strives to come up with a name that will fit the facts and will not have to be changed or revised with new knowledge.

When the word "perturbation" occurred to me, I ran to my dictionary and looked it up. What I read there gave me great excitement! One of the dictionary definitions of perturbation is *"a cause of mental disquietude."* I simply changed the adjective "a" to "the" and we have perturbation as *"the cause of mental disquietude."*

In the theory I am putting forth, a *perturbation is an isolable aspect of the thought field, which contains the necessary active and specific information to trigger highly specific negative emotions.*

Perturbation is used in physics and astronomy to indicate some kind of disturbance or difference from the norm. It has an implication of an almost random quality by this usage. However, the P in TFT is anything but random, for we know it contains highly precise information. The active information is so precise it controls and generates all of the consequences and activity of the various disturbing emotions. These consequences include the specific neural pathways used in various emotions, the chemical and hormonal factors released with each emotion, and the cognitive result of each of these. The concept of perturbation bridges the fields of psychology, physics, and biology.

New Facts For Psychology

Since we provide a simple algorithm for trauma, the reader can make observations and participate in what consists of revolutionary findings in clinical psychology. The algorithm for trauma, for example, will allow one to observe the following: We call these findings revolutionary in that nothing in conventional psychology could have predicted TFT nor can explain it. New concepts, such as thought field (TF) and perturbation (P) are required in order to comprehend what is taking place in this radically different treatment.

John, in the example above, when thinking about the trauma of ten years ago, illustrates what we call the tuning of a thought field. If the thought field has the isolable P contained within it, then there is an automatic generation of emotional upset when that thought field is tuned. When the simple algorithm or treatment is successfully administered, the thought no longer causes any upset. In most cases, this dramatic change holds over time. Sequelae such as nightmares, obsession, etc., also usually disappear.

Why Isolable?

We call the perturbation isolable because the therapy collapses it without affecting in any way the rest of the thought field. This is an extremely benevolent aspect of nature! Everything else in the thought field, such as the memory of the trauma and the details that once caused anguish, are still fully present but have lost all power to create upset. All information in the thought field remains the same after treatment except for the lack of upset. Obviously, therefore, the perturbation can be and is isolated from the rest of the thought field. To clearly see the meaning of "isolable" consider the dangerous "treatment" for fear of heights, which temporarily subsumes a perturbation but also removes other information, such as knowledge of the danger of heights, from the thought field (see the example of LSD, below).

Because of the common sequence of events in TFT—tuning—*upset*—therapy—tuning—*no upset*, I propose that an entity in the thought field, the perturbation, caused the upset. This entity is simply not functionally apparent after successful treatment.

Phobia Cure: "I Don't Believe It!"

Fear provides a good model to consider emotions. A phobia is a persistent fear that makes no sense. The person is afraid and knows he shouldn't be afraid, but can't help himself. Conventional psychologists believe it is impossible to actually cure a phobia (Adler 1993). Part of the definition of a phobia entails the notion of persistence—a phobia is a persistent fear. Joseph LeDoux (1994), an outstanding researcher on the brain, believes that when an emotional memory is put into the brain, it becomes indelible or non-removable.

Despite these common beliefs, TFT provides contrary facts. Such bold, robust, reproducible facts, previously unknown to psychology, demand new concepts in order to explain and comprehend the observed facts. TFT does not change the structure of the amygdala (part of brain), which would be required in the LeDoux theory. The reason conventional psychologists are having such a difficult time treating psychological problems is that they are looking in the wrong direction. The problem is not fundamentally in the brain or nervous system; it is in the thought field.

RESISTANCE TO THE NEW

Whenever revolutionary discoveries are made in science, initially there are overwhelming pressures to deny the facts. When that becomes impossible, the next stage of resistance is to attempt to force the new facts into the old explanations. Of course, science is naturally conservative and requires much evidence, but the present work puts powerful, reproducible evidence within immediate reach of any seriously interested person.

The attempts to suppress new, revolutionary findings are not only a function of the conservative nature of science, but also become placebos for minds that do not wish to do the necessary work required for radical change. Of course, if new facts could be adequately explained and integrated by old concepts, then a change of thought would not be necessary. The serious reader will discover that the radical new facts presented by TFT cannot even begin to be explained by the old and conventional concepts.

THE THOUGHT FIELD

The dictionary defines field as "a complex of forces that serve as causative agents in human behavior." The notion of a field is a most useful concept in modern science and the most fundamental concept in the TFT system. The thought field contains a great deal of information, but we select that which we consider central and pertinent to the generation of the negative emotions. It creates an imaginary, though quite real scaffold, upon which we may erect our explanatory notions. The term thought field is especially useful in work with conscious, mature humans who have a freedom and ability to choose to think about specific issues.

When working with animals or very young children who do not possess the ability to choose a thought, the term *perceptual field* is more appropriate. For example, when we wish to treat a young child or an animal, we cannot ask for specific thought tuning. The very young child and the animal must therefore be put into the situation, which causes upset before effective treatment is possible. I must emphasize that we always attempt to keep upset to an absolute minimum. Most conventional therapies encourage the person to be or to get upset. I believe suffering seeking behavior complicates treatment.

PERTURBATIONS

Due to the word "perturbation," some of my students have misunderstood the nature of this entity and equate it with "a disturbance in the thought field." This is quite incorrect; it controls the details of disturbance but is not itself a disturbance. The perturbation is anything but a random disturbance; it is rather a very carefully ordered (by nature) modulation in the thought field and is an exquisitely detailed and a highly specific signal. Perturbation is the proposed entity in the thought field that constitutes the most basic and fundamental cause (in a hierarchical chain of multiple causes) of *all* the negative emotions (such as fear, depression, anxiety, phobias, addictive urges, anger, trauma pain, etc).

Whether a fear is inherited, as in instinctive[1] or "prepared" fears such as snakes, heights, etc., or whether it occurs on the basis of a personal experience (as in trauma), we propose the fundamental causative unit of that fear is what we call the perturbation. The robust facts revealed by the treatments in TFT have forced me to posit these causative units.

I recognize that the negative emotions require an intact, conscious organism and involve hormonal, chemical, nervous, brain, and cognitive systems. The *fundamental* cause and triggering information that is primary, and in control of all the latter systems, is the perturbation. The perturbations are the aspect of the thought field that contains the specific triggering and controlling information for each negative emotion. If there is no perturbation in

---

[1] It is a common observation that phobias are not a random set, which would be expected if they were learned within the individual's lifetime. We propose that inherited phobias are learned by our ancient ancestors over millions of years and represent the common dangers (snakes and heights) that our ancient ancestors and evolutionary predecessors experienced.

the thought field, there is no negative emotion; conversely, if there is no negative emotion, then there is no perturbation in the thought field.

TFT causal diagnosis allows the therapist to palpably experience the perturbations in the thought field. The correctness of the TFT formulation that: *No perturbations = No disturbance* can become translated into a concrete experience. For the person limited to our algorithm level, this formulation provides a way to view exactly what happens in completely successful therapy.

Here are a few descriptive comments regarding the perturbation:

1. A perturbation is associated with a thought field.

2. Each perturbation in the thought field is associated with a specific energy meridian. The astonishing efficacy of TFT demands this notion. The meridian system is related to what is often (mistakenly) called the acupuncture meridians. Although this term identifies the correct category of energy meridians, the use of puncture refers merely to one method (insertion of needles) of addressing these meridians. Meridian is the more appropriate general term.

3. The functional presence of perturbations can be activated by normal development, biological process, or maturation. An example of perturbation's activation[2] by maturation is shown when the in-

---

[2] The inherited P is believed to have been present over eons in the form of Darwin's "invisible ink."

fant begins to crawl, which then engenders the ability to perceive converging lines of perspective. That, in turn, then engenders the fear of heights. The functional absence of perturbations (or, in other words, "Nature's therapy") may be observed when, with maturation, the child suddenly no longer has the automatic phobia of heights. Not all individuals pass through this higher maturation phase, but most do. I label the fear of heights of those who do not pass through this phase, *neotenous,* which is the common descriptive term in biology for a lack of complete development. The *atavistic* fear of heights refers to the re-introduction of the fear *after* it has been eliminated. The elimination can either be by maturation Nature's psychotherapy or by effective psychotherapy. The use of these biological terms in the psychological context has important utility.

4. Consider the fear of heights: All land-based chordates inherit as an instinct this fear. Land-based chordates are the animals that need protection from a fall. The fear is triggered when self-initiated movement begins. Self-initiated movement allows the organism to see the converging lines of perspective, which can signify height. Animals that are prevented from initiating their own movement are unable to perceive a declivity and hence can have no fear of heights. The fear ripens when the animal begins self-initiated movement.

LSD and Fear of Heights

LSD may be seen as "help" for the fear of heights, but, alas, it does more than subsume a perturbation. LSD not only temporarily subsumes a perturbation; it also removes one's knowledge about the danger of height. A number of young people have jumped out of windows under the influence of LSD. Biochemical assay labs use this information about the role of LSD in eliminating perturbations to test for the presence of LSD in blood.[3]

Baby chicks show fear (which indicates there are perturbations present) when placed next to an illusion of height. The illusion is used because it is just as effective as an actual height in generating fear and avoidance in a normal chick (or human). It prevents them from being hurt when they ignore it due to the influence of LSD. If the chick is injected with a drop of blood from an individual who has taken LSD, the chick will not show the normal fear (like humans) and walk over the illusion. In other words, the fear or phobia for heights is gone, indicating the perturbations have been subsumed. However, for humans to jump out of windows under LSD suggests the drug does more than eliminate the perturbations. It somehow eliminates the knowledge about the danger involved in height. John Lilly, who has studied dolphins, reports that dolphins show similar peculiar reactions in their response to depth when given LSD.

---

[3] I am grateful to Rupert Sheldrake for pointing out to me this interesting fact learned when he worked in such labs.

AUTOMATIC FEAR AND "NATURE'S THERAPY"

The Discovery Channel on television showed a marvelous brief piece on the hornbill bird. The African hornbill lays its eggs in the hollow of a tree and then seals it, except for a small opening for the feeding of the young. (Some species of hornbill seal up the mother as well.)

As the young hornbills mature, they have to chip open the protective covering on the opening to the nest in order to get out and fledge. In this film there were three hornbill youngsters laid and hatched just 48 hours apart. The behavior of these chicks was radically different due to the slight differences in their age. The oldest overcame his fear due to Nature's therapy, or maturation, of opening the closure and in order to get out of it began to chip away at the hole. The second oldest boldly attempted to stop the older chick from opening the hole and attempted to re-close it (droppings are used for this purpose). But, it is easier to open than close, and the older chick won out and escaped to fledge. The next older chick (#2) then patched up the hole. While the drama of hole opening was going on, the youngest chick (#3) was shivering with obvious fear in the far corner of the hollow (see drawing).

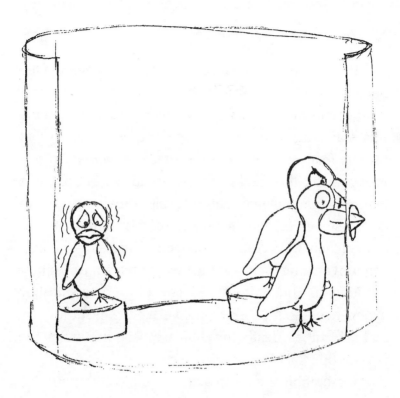

Just 48 hours difference in age cause the radical difference in the three distinct behaviors.

This is a very clear example of maturity or age having a direct effect on fear (or perturbations). Two days, or 48 hours, separate each chick. The two older chicks do not experience fear at the opening when they reach the appropriate age of maturity, but the youngest does. Four days after the first chick leaves and two days after the second chick leaves, the remaining chick has no fear. It opens up the hole to get out, fledge, and join its nestmates.

Natural Psychotherapy

In TFT terms, we believe that the perturbations in the perceptual field causing fear about leaving the nest, opening the hole, etc. was active until a certain age or maturity was reached. At that critical age, the perturbation that triggers fear, was subsumed naturally—*a natural psychotherapy*—and the chicks can go ahead with no or little fear. All young animals automatically experience fear in certain situations, and the purpose of this natural fear is to protect them from common dangers. If birds, for example, never overcame their fear they would remain in the nest too long and become easy victims of predators. If they experienced no fear, they would leave the nest too early and fall to their death. In both cases, Nature titrates the fear for optimal life.

Maturation, then, can activate (explode) a perturbation[4] or de-activate (implode) a perturbation. Successful therapy deactivates or subsumes a perturbation. We use the words subsumes and deactivate since the economy of Nature does not appear to squander such hard-won information contained within the perturbation by allowing a complete disappearance from the realm of potentiality. We say "hard-won" due to the death and injury of many members of the species and the suffering endured

---

[4] When a human infant begins to crawl, this aspect of development allows the perception of height to enter and the perturbation "explodes" at this time.

by survivors and witnesses to the traumas leading to the perturbations in thought or perceptual fields. In fact, Darwin considered that all established traits (physical and psychological) were fixed in a kind of "invisible ink" that could be revealed under certain stressful circumstances at any time.

The name given for such traits revived from the distant past is atavism. Heretofore, I have not found the commonly used terms atavism and neoteny used outside of biology, but I find them highly useful in understanding clinical psychological developmental issues.

CREATING PERTURBATIONS—OR, HOW DO P'S GET INTO A THOUGHT FIELD (TF)?

There are two main ways that P's can get into a thought field. One is through the experience of a trauma (not common) and the other is through inheritance. Perturbations can be introduced into thought fields (memory) in the laboratory by traumatizing animals, but this is cruel. The experiments of McDougall (1927) and successfully replicated by others (Crew, 1936, and Agar, Drummond, and Tiegs, 1942) show that traumatic information is encoded and inherited by future generations of the species, i.e., *it is not limited* to the offspring of those who experienced the trauma (see Sheldrake). The whole species appears to encode and "remember" (in the form of perturbations in the thought field) commonly occurring traumas. The trigger for and detailed guiding and specific information for the disturbing emotion connected with the trauma is laid down in the form of perturbations. One can observe, both in humans and animals, that perturbations are introduced through traumatic experiences.

The aspects of trauma that we call obsession, reliving, nightmares, rumination, etc. are the means Nature has established through natural selection to record, reinforce, and imprint vital information in reality. See Sheldrake (1989) for a scientific hypothesis that which can account for the inheritance of such information.

The following interesting report is by experimental psychologist Neal Miller (1995):

> [In] an early experiment of mine (Miller, 1951), I trained an individual to show a discriminated, conditioned galvanic skin response indicating fear of the symbol T, presented to him and followed by an electric shock, but not of the symbol 4, presented without shock. When presented with a series of dots and told to think 4 to the first one and T to the next, and so on, *the fear transferred from the overt cues to the thoughts...* [my emphasis]." (p. 909) One may see from this how a P gets into the thoughts, or as I would say, the thought field.

When we treat an attuned thought field, it could be said we are directly treating the original fear or other upsetting association. A test is to then expose the successfully treated client to an actual situation and see what happens. The reason "*a* test" rather than "*the* test" is that it is well known in clinical TFT work that a cure, even a *complete* cure, may be undone. This is known to occur in TFT when the client has sensitivities to certain "toxins." (M. Miller, 1996)

Homeostasis Creates Complexity

The exposure to or ingestion of such selective toxins (e.g., nicotine, wheat, etc.) will, in a small number of cases, predictably regenerate or recreate the problem. It is speculated that such regeneration is a function of homeostasis and in general may operate to prevent a toxin from leading into unlimited severity by translating it into a form of complexity instead; it spreads the risk around the organism. Homeostasis, as one scientist put it, makes potentially deadly problems more complex rather than deadly. The translation of toxins into complexity can save one's life.

The first thing I discovered when doing this work was that it is critical *what the patient thinks about during diagnosis and treatment.* To give it a name more specifically than the rather vague "what is thought about," the term thought field was introduced. At that time (1979), I wrote that the process was somewhat like tuning into a particular radio station. Tune to a different station and you get completely different information. In fact, it is this dynamic, changing characteristic of the thought field that is distinctive to the field of clinical psychology and TFT and gives it more potential complexity than other fields of healing. A dentist or an acupuncturist, for example, does not require the patient to think about anything in particular in order to treat a complaint. Professions other than clinical psychology are addressing what I call the more "inertial laden," or physical aspects, of a person. It is because of the low inertia of the P that TFT therapy is so rapid.

Most psychologists have been aware for years that specific thoughts have a definite impact on a person. Indeed, this very idea forms a fundamental basis of clinical psychology. Out of the vast realm of possible conscious and subconscious thoughts, what the person is aware of, or tuned in to, at a particular time can and usually does have a profound effect on the total being especially if the thought field has active perturbations. Different TF's have different P's and this is one of the major facts that is responsible for my therapy being so powerful. My causal diagnosis procedure allows one to reveal the specific perturbations in any one of an almost infinite number of TF's.

Very young children and animals of course are not able to produce a particular thought field on demand. In animal research the thought field is controlled through the situation; e.g., having a pigeon "think about food" by starving him; having a rat "think about danger or pain" by shocking it. Here the thought fields or perceptual fields are imposed.

If you have any of my video demonstration tapes, a particularly good example of what I mean by thought field tuning is illustrated by the woman on the national television show *Evening Magazine*. She had been unable to drive on freeways or over bridges for 18 years.[5] You can see her shift from an easygoing and relaxed manner into a severe anxiety state when she tunes into the driving problem and breaks down with emotion.

---

[5] This example may be seen on the videotape called "Introduction to TFT" (LaQuinta, CA).

She is a good example of what we are discussing because her emotions flow smoothly, she is not obstructed, repressed, or blocked on awareness of how disturbing this problem can be. Often, with other people, especially men, we would have to inquire as to how they feel. The severely repressed individual is *aware* of feeling nothing until the emotion becomes overwhelming in an actual situation.

The severely repressed individual can be diagnosed and treated as easily as the non-repressed person due to the fact that *the perturbations are manifest in the thought field regardless of the level of awareness.* The manifestation of the perturbations when a perturbed thought field is attuned provides the basis for our unique causal diagnostic system. This exciting procedure actually allows the person trained in causal diagnosis to palpate and address the specific perturbations, which are causing any particular problem.

DISTINGUISHING PERTURBATIONS IN THOUGHT FIELD AND MEMORY

The powerful effect of TFT necessitates the identification of a specific aspect of the thought field as particularly significant. What might we call this aspect? Some psychologists believe that effective psychotherapy treatment removes a memory. Although the term "memory" has some relevance in this context, it is too broad a term to be meaningful in the therapy context and is very misleading. The thought field is more similar to memory as we use the term. It seems necessary to distinguish a particular aspect of the thought field—the aspect that is present prior to therapy (or maturation) and absent after. The term memory in this context simply does not identify this critical aspect but includes too much. We find, for example, after treating severe traumas, that the memory of the trauma is still perfectly intact though all trace of upset is gone. Obviously some portion of the thought field is different after successful therapy—the difference is the absence of the entity I call the perturbation.

We have overwhelming evidence, especially apparent in our trauma treatments, to indicate that the global memory of a trauma is in no way affected by the treatment. If anything, memory of the traumatic incident may even become clearer with the removal of the devastating and disruptive emotions that typically accompany traumatic incidents. Such emotions typically prevent one from looking clearly at terribly traumatic events because the pain, due to the P is unbearable.

Clearly, what one thinks about has an effect on the person. This fact delineates the thought field. The typical disturbed client gets quite upset when tuning into the thought field of any intense problem. When a formerly very disturbed person thinks about a problem after successful treatment, with no apparent discomfort, there must be some features in the thought field that have changed *after* the treatment. Since there is no upsetting emotion where formerly there was a quite upsetting emotion, we posit that the fundamental cause of that emotion, the entity we call a perturbation, has been collapsed with successful therapy.

It does not matter whether a perturbation is established from experience, knowledge, or given through a different means of heredity than the genes, e.g., by the past collective experiences of paleo-ancestors (in the group soul, collective unconscious or the morphic fields). *The P is the direct and fundamental local container, transmitter and transposer of negative emotions.* The appropriateness or inappropriateness of the emotion is irrelevant. Whether appropriate or inappropriate, the negative emotion is always fundamentally caused by the presence of a perturbation in a thought field. A perturbation evolves as a relationship between the body and the mind. It appears to be a structural entity with meaning; that is, it conveys emotional meaning to an event. The meaning contained in a perturbation(s) is usually quite dramatic.

THOUGHT FIELD (TF)

The thought field is important in treatment because of the development of consciousness. Part of this development in humans is that a choice is possible, which is critical in treatment, and allows one to *attune* a particular thought field. Our work shows that attunement is immediate and requires no special effort and *no obvious time period.* This was surprising to me. I used to give a client some time to "get into" a particular thought, but we have evidence to show that the thought field is immediately present.

The no-obvious-time requirement is shown by the fact that perturbations appear instantly (as revealed in diagnosis) the moment the intention to tune is formed. Time may be required before the person is *aware* of the emotional impact of tuning, but that is quite a separate issue.

Attunement, along with its consequent suffering, appears to be an end in itself in the emotional reliving kind of exposure therapy. However, this suffering does not result in the automatic elimination of perturbations. One "benefit" that emotional reliving as a therapy might have seems similar to that of hitting oneself on the head with a hammer because it feels so good when it is stopped.

A virtual thought field is not tuned. One may have an unlimited number of thought fields with perturbations, but they cause no negative emotion unless tuned. Tuning, of course, may be by choice or imposed by a situation or obsession.

All disturbed emotions, such as anger, anxiety, depression, addictive urge, and trauma have perturbations in common. The concept of perturbation thus unifies all the negative or disturbing emotions through the notion of a proposed common cause. The perturbation is the container of the necessary information to trigger specific negative emotional reactions.

In the case of phobias, clearly the perturbations are in some sort of informational flow from the past (millions of years) into the present. Phobias persist over millennia, even useless phobias for the modern city-dwelling person, such as fear of snakes. Why don't phobias dissipate or disappear? The flow of information is in both directions—from the past and toward the future—but there is little energy incentive for phobias to dissipate with time.

Fish living in caves, for example, lose their non-functional eyes and the energy that would be taken to construct and maintain an eye is available for other organs and survival issues. The energy requirement of the information in the perturbations (due to lower inertia) seems to persist over time. A partially relevant analogy here is an audiotape: the tape itself is inertial laden while the information on the tape (the electromagnetic pattern) is very low in inertia. This low-inertia (mass) we believe, is why it is so relatively easy (when one knows the proper codings) to eliminate phobias and traumas.

This flow of information can explain how a common trauma at one time may become an inherited phobia later in time. McDougall's careful research (1927) is a clear indication of this fascinating and life-protecting function and demonstrates the interesting fact that such information is passed on to future members of the species. McDougall's work was largely ignored since there was no known *genetic* means of transmission of such information. Rupert Sheldrake (1987, 1989) provides a coherent theoretical and non-genetic basis for such transmission, as does Jung's notion of the "collective unconscious." The traumas experienced by McDougall's rats caused phobias in future generations.

The relatively simple perturbation (after the P code of Nature is understood and used in psychotherapy) communicates the *emotionally* significant information regarding phobias. It seems to generate fear when associated with an appropriate sign stimulus, such as perception in the fear of heights. The infant, therefore, who shows a fear when confronted with the perception of height, does not need to understand height, laws of gravity, falling, or even the notion of danger or harm, or getting hurt. The infant is automatically afraid[6] when confronted with this perception, which consists of being proximal to downward-converging lines. Even the close-bonded and highly trusted mother cannot get the infant to go on the glass when the infant is confronted with the perception of height (Gibson and Walk, 1960). Most individuals grow out of this automatic intense fear, but some do not. Those who do not are called acrophobes.

I believe this perturbation became established with the perception of height, associated with trauma of personal hurt and pain as well as hurt and pain of loved ones, over millions of years, and is transmitted to future generations as McDougall and others (as interpreted by Sheldrake) have demonstrated. Genetics cannot adequately account for the means of transmission. It requires some extra-chemical means such as morphic resonance as Sheldrake hypothesizes (Sheldrake, 1981).

After this fear is established and serves its protective function, it disappears in the more developed animals or humans. The appearance and common disappearance of the fear may be compared to the maturation-based fear and its natural "cure" that occurs in the previously mentioned hornbill. A perturbation comes into being, and is then, after a time, naturally collapsed or subsumed. This

---

6   This fear information is transmitted to other members of the species even though there is no genetic connection and is "broadcast" all over the universe (Sheldrake).

may happen almost instantly when a certain maturation level is achieved. TFT as a treatment works rapidly also, since we believe we are using nature's psychotherapy and a similar process would therefore be expected.

The rapid elimination of perturbations when no longer needed is a hallmark of nature. It has been observed by many scientists, beginning with Liebnez and Maupertuis (Young, 1979), that nature shows an interesting, even intelligent economy. The formal name for this fact is commonly called The Least Action Principle or the Variation Principle. The founder of the fundamental discovery in quantum physics, Max Planck, named his basic discovery, the *quantum of action*, after the Least Action principle. TFT, along this line, with its remarkable speed and effectiveness, could be considered a Least Action therapy. There are valid specific reasons why therapy is so rapid and effective. The most obvious is the fact that psychological problems are not grounded in the actual network of neurons, the DNA or the brain.

ANTICIPATORY ANXIETY

Anticipatory anxiety is often used as a descriptive term in work with phobic or anxiety clients. It appears to be a term suggesting or implying the client has a choice to not become disturbed prior to an actual situation.

I take issue with this notion. Anticipatory anxiety is nothing more than tuning into a perturbed thought field. This experience is evidence that the person needs effective (TFT) therapy.

If a thought field contains perturbations resulting in intense emotions, the attunement of this thought field will cause upsetting or distressing emotion. This is no more than the usual demonstration of the fact that perturbations are present and reflects the commonplace observation in our system that a perturbed thought field will result in upsetting emotions. And of course, if there are no perturbations, the treated person will show no disturbing emotion. I see, therefore, no special significance to the term "anticipatory anxiety" and believe the notion is misleading. All anxiety, whether anticipatory or in a particular situation, is simply due to the presence of perturbations in the thought field.

There are those whose interest in working with people is more in the realm of values and philosophical beliefs. It is my belief that many therapists drifted into this realm because they learned that they actually could not offer much actual help for psychological problems. Some of them, such as Rollo May, would go even further to criticize and denigrate the removal of symptoms. The position of such therapists would become more convincing if they learned some of the modern power therapies and *still* maintained their point of view. This point seems somewhat similar to my experience many years ago in looking at the works of Van Gogh. I took a fresh interest in his work when I came across some of his old sketches that showed me he could really draw very well. Therefore, I took a new look at his later and more well-known works, since I knew that he was *choosing* to paint the way he did and that it was not due to a limitation in skill.

Only therapists who have achieved the rare, almost unheard of skill to rapidly eliminate disturbing symptoms are entitled to be critical of the process.

HEALING DATA

However, TFT is now being successfully applied to many problems other than just psychological. A growing number of physicians, naturopaths, chiropractors, massage therapists, acupuncturists and other healing professionals are successfully using TFT to help many problems. Our work appears to be outgrowing the term perturbation. It is clear that causal diagnosis yields a code—a code which when carried out will typically eliminate a problem. As medical and other problems are being successfully addressed with this work, a term that can accurately denote the process of therapy is needed.

I have been greatly impressed with the work of cybernetician David Foster, author of two powerful books, *The Intelligent Universe* and *The Philosophical Scientists*. He has designed a number of programs allowing various factories to be run by computer. Foster sees a deep analogy between the universe, molecular biology and information theory. Many of the early 20th-century scientists, before they were made busy making weapons for a warring world, were very much impressed with the idea that as Arthur Eddington put it: "The stuff of the world is mind stuff [or data]." (Foster, 1975, p. 41)

Developments in molecular biology appear to closely approximate the work of the information theorist, or computer programmer. "The result of this to the molecular biologist who has to unfathom the further secrets is that he now has no option but to treat his nucleic acids as data complexes and to use the methods of the information theorist as to 'code cracking.' A DNA molecule is seen as a piece of coding."

Foster's works resonated strongly with my own work. As my discoveries became more obvious and successful, it became clear what I call causal diagnosis was the pursuit of the specific code needed to correct a problem. My discoveries of rather simple algorithms with which one may rapidly eliminate various problems has evidently blinded some who take the algorithms as a given. They forget that before causal diagnosis there were no such algorithms. The algorithms simply represent codes I discovered in nature, which have startling success rates. Before causal diagnosis there were no such codes.

The need for correct codes is made crystal clear when we encounter a complex case where the algorithm will not help. Here a series of codes are revealed by sophisticated causal diagnosis, which will then help a complex case. As I have made more discoveries over the last two decades, my success rate has been gradually increasing and getting very close to perfection. This work is now on a par with hard science, physics and chemistry. We are no longer floundering in the wispy world of social science.

Foster makes it very clear that data (knowledge, information) is the link between body and mind. My concept of perturbation is clearly such a link. As mentioned, however, the perturbation, though ideal as a cause of psychological problems is wanting as we expand to help many other problems. A new term is needed.

The term I have chosen as the broader and more precisely accurate term in our expanding context is *healing data*. It seems very clear that my discoveries have identified controls for the natural healing system. It is clear this system, just as in molecular biology, consists of codes. In the healing system the codes are composed from a correct series of acupuncture points, otherwise known as data.

Foster (1975) presents a strong case, that everything in the universe is composed of data, specific data.

> The idea that solid tangible matter is also intrinsically data is not so obvious. But, in 1927 Louis de Broglie showed that solid matter could equally be considered as a wave or vibration system, and the earlier Quantum Theory of Max Planck had similarly accounted for the structure of the atom in terms of the wave motions of orbital electrons. The totality of these findings was that the only way of describing matter in a fundamental sense was by means of mathematical equations rather than as an agglomerate of microscopical billiard balls, and this is why Professor Eddington[7] in 1927 or so began to suspect that "the stuff of the world is mind stuff," albeit rather mathematical mind stuff. (p. 40).

In 1965, Foster demonstrated mathematically to the British Association meeting in Dundee, that Planck's constant was the "ultimate unit of information" and the Cosmic Binary digit (1975, p. 38). The Mendeleev table in

---

[7] Eddington was the first scientist to prove Einstein correct.

chemistry shows about 100 chemical elements, which differ in specific ways, and Foster proposes that this is Nature's complex alphabet from which the world—the universe—is constructed. It is impossible to do justice to the two books of Foster in a brief manner and therefore, the serious student should obtain these books and devote study to them.

Cybernetics is Foster's specialty. The term was introduced years earlier by Norbert Wiener and means in Greek "the art of the steersman." It refers to control. Control in TFT, in our broadened context, is control of the healing system. The basic objects, which govern control, are now called healing data (HD). Our causal diagnoses reveal the healing data in the correct order in order to eliminate a problem. Our term HD is more precise for general problems than is the more limited term of perturbation.

CHAPTER 13

EMOTIONAL CONTROL SYSTEM

The all-or-nothing nature of nerve action can thus be understood as simply another instance, in this case in higher organisms, of the quantum leap so firmly established in the atomic and molecular realms. Now, since control, conscious or unconscious, employs nerve action, and nerve action proceeds by quantum jumps, we may deduce that control in life processes proceeds by quantum jumps—and that the terminal point in the chain of command is the quantum of action.

Arthur M. Young

To begin to understand control, let's start with the dictionary definition:

To exercise restraining or directing influence over, to have power over, an act or instance of controlling, power or authority to guide or manage; skill in the use of a tool, instrument, or technique; To eliminate or prevent the spread of: to control a forest fire [or we would say "panic"]; the act or power of controlling; regulation, domination, or command; a device for regulating or guiding a machine; a coordinated arrangement of control devices; prevention of the flourishing or spread of something undesirable; Synonym: manage, govern, rule, restrain; mastery.

THERAPY PROGRESSES BY QUANTUM JUMPS

One of the robust findings regarding TFT is that the therapy progresses in quantum-type leaps. That is, the person whose problem starts off at an upset (SUD) level of 10 will show a distinct pattern in the manner in which progress occurs. In the first phase of the treatment, administering the majors, typically results in a definite sudden reduction from a 10 to a 7; the gamut series will typically bring the problem down to a 4 and the repeat of the majors will usually move the person to a 1. The interesting thing about this progress, which usually takes place within minutes, is that the person jumps from one level to the next without passing through the intermediate levels of experiencing the problem. This pattern goes against not only conventional psychological experience but against the reasonable expectations of the client. But, this result fits observations in quantum physics.

It is stunning enough that our unusual therapy has the power to eliminate problems as completely as it does, but it is even more stunning that the nature of the change takes place by large jumps. Conventional expectations or commonsense reality would lead one to expect a gradual change, under the best of circumstances, over a period of months or years. The nature and manner of this change is similar to quantum theory.

In discussing some of the stunning facts re quantum theory, physicist David Peat (1990) describes the mystery of the quantum jump:

> Quantum theory makes yet another radical break with our commonsense approach to reality; not only does a quantum particle seem to be in two different places at the same time—it can also move between two points without ever occupying the intermedi-ate space between.../Q]uantum theory parts com-pany with everyday analogies.... In place of a continuous change is a discontinuous leap.... Quan-tum theorists call this discontinuous transition the quantum jump. " (pp. 13-15)

Many physicists are contributing to an understand-ing of consciousness (see Penrose, Goswami, Bohm [1990], and Stapp.) Goswami, states: "[T]here is plenty of evidence of discontinuity—quantum jumps—in mental phe-nomena, especially in the phenomenon of creativity

(p. 163)." He goes on: "What we call the mind consists of objects that are akin to the objects of submicroscopic matter and that obey rules similar to those of quantum mechanics (p. 167)."

I had the pleasure of meeting Professor Goswami when we each presented at a Behavioral Medicine Conference a few years ago. The quantum jumps I reported (and demonstrated at this conference) in my therapy seemed perfectly natural to him.

Henry Stapp is a leading quantum theorist and in the glossary of his book *Mind Matter and Quantum Mechanics* (1993) he describes "event": "A quantum event is the sudden change of the quantum state from one form to another. This event is also called the quantum jump, the collapse of the wave function, or the reduction of the wave packet." (p. 235)

Stapp is very impressed with William James, the American psychologist of the last century, for James foresaw, even before quantum theory, that classical physics was unsuitable for contributing to an understanding of the mind.

In a very interesting addition, Stapp's discussion of a "metastable" condition could well serve as a model for my causal diagnosis procedures. He says:

> In this situation, there is a...change of the observable macroscopic state of the device from one metastable configuration to another [due to]...a measuring device that is being used to measure some property of an atomic-sized quantum system.... The de-

vice must be in a state of unstable[1] equilibrium, so that a small signal from the atomic-sized system can trigger a chain of events leading to a change of certain observable features of the device.

Actually, if one is scientifically oriented, and hopes ultimately to find a physical basis for mind, it should be clear that if there is a physical or material basis for mind, it must accord with the most advanced understanding of matter which is, quantum theory.

Arthur M. Young states that the kind of quantum jumps to which I refer is *"typical of control in life processes."* Young (1980) has more to say about such control systems than any writer I have come across so far, and indeed he chides conventional physics for leaving out the third derivative,[2] which is *control.*

Some critics of the quantum of action, emphasizing the extremely small amount of energy available, have said the quantum of action does not have enough energy to

---

[1] Early designers of aircraft had *stable equilibrium* built into their models. It is interesting to observe that the Wright brothers, unlike their competitors, and at a cost of an increased risk of crashing, wanted their aircraft to be in an *unstable* equilibrium in order that it could be *controlled.* Not only did the Wright brothers invent the first self-powered aircraft, they invented the methods of control of such an aircraft, which were unknown at the time. Arthur Young, who invented the Bell helicopter, discovered important principles of *control* for this newer aircraft.

[2] Through his development of the calculus, Isaac Newton introduced the two derivatives, velocity and acceleration, which provided the basis for the science of motion. Young (1990) maintains that science unfortunately excludes the third derivative, which is control. Engineers use control but science neglects it. The third derivative provides the basis for the science of cybernetics (helmsman or control).

lift a finger. Young points out the quantum of action *does not have to lift anything*. When you push an elevator button you do not lift the elevator—a hierarchical series of electrical and mechanical devices do this work. You make the decision[3] to push the button, you push it and what follows is a beautiful illustration of how life processes work if everything is functioning smoothly (when there is no illness or significant relevant psychological problem present). Issues at the headquarters (control) level require no more than a minuscule amount of energy; typically just enough to move an electron, which then has a cascading effect on the rest of the system. We don't need to lift the elevator; we merely push the button. This is a superb metaphor for how life processes work. When you drive a car you exert very little effort or energy, especially today with power steering, power brakes, etc. A very slight pressure on the steering wheel allows you to control a car that weighs over a ton and a half or allows the pilot of a 747 aircraft to control that huge mass with very little effort.

Control systems involve hierarchies of systems. At the top of the system is a device requiring the smallest pressure or energy such as the steering wheel of a car. This device is in turn connected to a number of other systems, which finally result in the desired effect. Engineers specialize in building control systems into machinery so that a human can exert control with a minimum of energy. Machines would be worthless if they required more energy to operate than they deliver.

---

[3] Young states that the quantum of action *is* decision.

LIFE AND CONTROL SYSTEMS

Biology has control systems built into life beginning at the stage of one-celled animals. Movement of amoebae is done in the simple, clever way of changing its shape. Of course, intake of food and oxygen and expulsion of waste products are all controlled largely by automated processes. Automated or instinctual in life process means that at one time it required some sort of what we must call conscious effort; then later, with much practice, the activity became automatic—i.e., done without effort or thought given to it. When you first learned to drive a car you had to pay attention to a number of details to which you give no conscious thought today. The driving process has become so instinctual that you can carry on a conversation while driving.

Many control systems operate by what we call instinct, which in general terms refers to the fact that no conscious effort is required for the operation of the control system. There seems no question that many instincts are inherited, but the precise manner in which this inheritance takes place is not clear at this time. Though most people assume heredity must be genetic, it is not likely that exquisitely detailed psychological information is contained in DNA or the genes. No one has ever shown how that could be likely or even possible. I agree with Rupert Sheldrake when he notes that brains and genes are overrated.

THE CONTROL SYSTEM FOR THE NEGATIVE EMOTIONS

David Foster, in *The Philosophical Scientists* (1985), reviews the major discoveries of physics in this century. He makes the astonishing pronouncement:

> All the major developments in physics in this century have been of mystical origin, with the outcome generally being some new mathematical formulae. If one considers the mystical experiences of the great pioneering scientists, then in each case one can deduce that they experienced mystical revelation. One might quote:
>
> Planck and quantum theory
> Einstein and relativity theory
> DeBroglie and matter-wave mechanics
> Schrodinger and wave mechanics
> Heisenberg and the uncertainty principle
> Pauli and the exclusion principle.
>
> Not one of these was reasonable or common sense, but all were true and they worked.[4] (p. 147)

Many mathematical discoveries appear to come into being through some kind of mystical intuition. Foster (1985) cites Henri Poincaire, who found the solution to a difficult problem as he put his foot on the step of an omni-

---

[4] It is known that they worked through the application of scientific tests. "Worked" in this context means that these "mystical" developments were shown to articulate with reality. The reader, can test my claims, for example, by trying the procedure on people and see for themselves how TFT works in reality.

bus. The solution came to him in an instant with no effort and no thought. He knew instantly or recognized that the solution was correct even though he had no time to check it out in his mind and did not do so until he returned from whence he came. Poincaire went through the proving routine for "conscience's sake" and not because he needed to verify the correctness. It is often written that the foundation of organic chemistry, the ring of six carbon atoms, came to August von Kekule in his dream of a snake that seized its own tail.

Gantum Nair (1996) tells about a group of scientists who are attempting to program computers in a manner that mimics the way Nature solves problems, which is usually quite anti-intuitive or anti-common sense. David Liddle is quoted regarding nature: "Her reckless and random ways" are valued. "[H]umans rely on logical processes, they consider a fairly narrow range of solutions, he argues; nature, on the other hand, takes a sprawling trial and error approach that tests many more potential solutions." (p. A1) Nair adds: "Our view of computer science is rational, mechanistic. But nature winds up doing things in a way we'd never think of, Mr. Liddle says." (p. A1) This same article points out a common finding in science that when different specialties are cross-pollinated they sometimes arrive at findings similar to Nature's. TFT was developed when my background in clinical psychology was cross-pollinated with a special finding in the field of the chiropractic subspecialty of Applied Kinesiology (Walther) and the meridians of acupuncture.

TFT Is Nature's Therapy

The reason TFT encounters the ubiquitous apex problem, and why most therapists assume TFT cannot possibly work, and why even some of those who successfully use it remain skeptical, is that TFT does not follow a reasonable, rationally derived (to the conventional mind) program. Nature was studied firsthand and TFT revealed itself. This is why the therapy appears so peculiar to most people, especially those conversant with conventional psychology. TFT does not make sense from the conventional point of view; however, it is *nature's own therapy.* It is without doubt the most powerful, effective therapy of all time. We are tapping into nature's healing system.

Of course, the therapy is peculiar and unfamiliar; it appears to make no sense whatsoever. *However, no other therapy can come close to the power and range of this approach.* You can test this using the algorithm provided for trauma.

TFT, this peculiar, non-logical therapy, was first discovered to be highly successful with phobias. Later, as a result of additional discoveries I found it to be a powerful predictable treatment for trauma. As new discoveries were made, I found TFT to be an equally effective treatment for addiction. In the majority of cases TFT can eliminate all traces of the additive urge and all symptoms of withdrawal, even for heroin, in most addicts within minutes. Further discoveries found that TFT was a powerful treatment for depression, anger, jealousy, obsession, and anxiety and in fact, for any negative emotion and/or stress. The extension of TFT into all these new areas with such a predictably high success rate allows us to state with considerable confidence that the control system for the negative emotions has been discovered. All the negative emotions, in the vast majority of cases (98%) can now be rapidly and successfully treated with properly administered TFT.

Predictability and extraordinary success rates due to our diagnostic procedures allow us to make this claim. We believe when we diagnose the perturbations at the root of a psychological problem or negative emotion, we are revealing the code existing within nature that determines, at the most fundamental level, the negative emotions.

The control system for the negative emotions has been in place for many millions of years, but no one knew where to look for it. Most efforts have been misplaced and the searches are looking in the wrong direction, such as the amygdala of the brain (LeDoux 1994, 1995) or the chemical approach so common today. These are feeble attempts to change the disturbing emotions. The chemical approach commonly leads to addictions to drugs and also to potentially dangerous side effects. We are obviously indirectly changing the chemistry of the system with this approach, but in a perfectly natural and harmless manner. With successful treatment, the chemistry is balanced without the risk of drugs.

DISORDERS AND ENTROPY

The Second Law of Thermodynamics—the law that entropy always increases—is perhaps the most robust law in science. Entropy is disorder, the tendency for everything to move toward disorder. "Almost all physical processes are wayward and subjected to shuffling and disorder...." (Foster, p. 105) This law is associated with thermodynamics because it is mainly used to refer to the motion of atoms in gases under the influence of heat but can refer to a deck of cards, information, or even life processes. In this view, death is complete entropy. But illness, disease, and disorder can be viewed as entropy of a lesser degree than the complete entropy of death. Foster notes that shuffling cards involves no consciousness but sorting cards into their suits and number does involve consciousness.

Foster gives a good explanation of entropy using a deck of playing cards. They come from the store ordered in their four suits and sequences.

> If we now shuffle the cards then we increase their entropy, their state of random disorder, until they come into a state where no further shuffling can increase the random disorder, in which case we have reached maximum entropy.... Two matters should be noted: 1. Entropy can be reduced by *conscious sorting*.... A conscious sorting entity can reduce entropy and reverse the Second Law of Thermodynamics. 2. The shuffling of the card pack essentially takes place in a state of absent-mindedness, i.e., *the mental opposite* of the conscious sorting of (1) above.

When we treat a person with TFT, we are restoring order to the disorder or reducing the entropy. As Foster put it, "all physical systems are subject to disorder," but he adds, *"they can only be controlled by a programme which is specific."* Our work with the control system, the specifics of which are revealed by our causal diagnosis, strongly supports the specific nature of a treatment required to restore order. The causal diagnoses reveal the specific codes needed to restore order. Many practitioners of my work at the algorithm (the lowest level) are not aware that the codes used in successful algorithms were revealed by causal diagnosis. As David Bohm once said in a radio interview, if there were no order to the disorder, no help would be possible.

With knowledge of the codes in nature, one can control or eliminate the negative emotions. Much human suffering is now no longer necessary. In a very real sense we can now put Humpty Dumpty together again, or as Macbeth expressed it, we can *"pluck from the mind a rooted sorrow."*

CHAPTER 14

MEMORY

The memory is no more in the brain than the picture coming from a television studio is in the television receiver.

Rupert Sheldrake

Many experts in the field of trauma seem to believe the problem in trauma is in the memory of the event. Some experts are attempting to develop drugs that will obliterate or impair the memory of a trauma. I believe this is terribly misguided. It is easy to understand why they think this because the memory is what appears to be causing the problem. However, my work teaches us clearly that the problem is not at all in the memory. How do I know? When you do the simple treatment for trauma provided in this book, please observe the following. Immediately upon finishing the treatment you will see clearly the person, who had experienced extreme suffering before treatment, will maintain a perfectly clear memory of the incident without that memory causing any upset.

The facts of TFT appear to lend support to Sheldrake's notion as quoted. Why? If the fundamental information causing disturbed emotions were in the hard wiring of the brain or in the structure of the amygdala, it could not possibly be eradicated or collapsed so quickly as we regularly do in TFT. Joseph LeDoux's (1994, 1995) notion of indelibility, which states that trauma is indelibly imprinted in the brain, is supported by conventional psychotherapy which readily admits (Adler, 1993) their treatments cannot be permanent and are easily undone. This notion is quite convincingly toppled by TFT.

The dictionary defines memory as:

> The power or process of reproducing or recalling what has been learned and retained especially through associative mechanisms; persistent modification of structure or behavior resulting from an organism's activity or experience; the store of things learned and retained as evidenced by recall and recognition of an image or impression of someone or something remembered; the time within which past events can be or are remembered.

A good many therapists and research scientists see effective psychotherapy as somehow doing something to the "memory"; for example, if a trauma is treated successfully the therapist might report that the memory of the trauma has been eradicated. Such use of the omnibus term memory in a therapy context creates a number of confusing problems and we have recommendations concerning this common usage.

THERAPY AND MEMORY

Regarding therapy changing a memory, one must consider the following relevant facts:

1. When TFT cures the nightmares and pain of trauma, the person's memory of the trauma appears to be totally unaffected. If anything the memory may be even clearer due to the complete lack of emotional disturbance now associated with the memory. A person who is not emotionally shaken to the core is more able to see the facts relevant to the traumatic incident more clearly.

2. If a person is traumatized by the loss of someone close, even a precious child, the successfully treated person does not "forget" the child is gone.

WHERE ARE MEMORIES STORED?

Aristotle introduced the idea that memory is like a sealing wax impression. Descartes introduced the idea memories were stored in the nervous system. The conventional view today is that memory traces are stored in the synapses of the nerves and somehow stored inside the brain. Some believe they are stored as molecules and some that they are dependent upon electrical vibrations. All believe memories are stored in the brain as patterns of some kind. If these notions were correct, it would mean we would have to have vast memories stored within our brains (Ian Marshall, 1989), requiring more synapses and nerves, by far, than are available.

There is a great deal of research available that raises certain questions, especially from Lashley (1950). He trained monkeys how to open a complex latch on a door. In an effort to find out where memories are stored, he systematically began removing portions of brain. He found that he could remove up to 50% of the brain, top, left, right, etc., and they could still open the latch. He also found rats could learn mazes and he could remove up to 70% of the brain and they still could run the maze successfully. If he removed the whole brain they couldn't do it anymore (Sheldrake, 1981). No matter *where* he cut, the monkey, after time would remember the trick, unless too much of the brain was destroyed.

Lashley's student, Karl Pribram, developed the theory that memory is stored throughout the brain in what are called interference patterns, like a hologram, i.e., it is not located in any particular region, but is everywhere throughout the whole brain. The main evidence in favor of this theory, according to Sheldrake (1990), is that so far no one has been able to find localized memory traces. Therefore, memory must not be localized and must be something like a hologram. But this assumes, of course, the memories must be in the brain.

Only Sheldrake's theory considers the possibility that memory is not stored in the brain at all. This is an alternative way of explaining why no one can find localized traces of memory within brains. He wrote: "If the memories are not in the brain, then it is not surprising no one has been able to find them, despite decades of intensive effort, the expenditure of hundreds of millions of dollars, and the destruction of tens of thousands of unfortunate animals."

No one has yet succeeded in locating any of these hypothetical memory traces. No one has even been able to say of what they might consist. For some time it was thought RNA molecules might be an answer, but that theory was dropped due to a lack of evidence. For the synapse theory to be an adequate explanation, the synapses would have to be extraordinarily stable, but in fact they are changing continually. This is a big problem and the molecular biologists do not have an answer for this objection.

Logical Problem

Philosophers have pointed out that, if you have a memory store, then you must have a retrieval system that can go to the store and take out the right memories. In order to recognize the memory it must itself have a memory and then one gets into an infinite regress that each retrieval system must have a retrieval system, etc. This introduces a fundamental, serious criticism of the logic of memory storage and traces being in the brain. But, as Sheldrake (1990) points out, despite all these obvious shortcomings, most experts continue to believe memories are stored in the brain. Most people believe this, saying, "Memory must be in the brain, for if it were not in the brain where else could it be?" The lack of evidence and the logical problem does not matter.

Sheldrake proposes that memory involves tuning into the past. The difficult facts seem more intelligible when seen from this point of view.

Penfield (1975) gave mild electric shocks to the brains of patients and they experienced vivid memories. At first Penfield suggested this proved memories were in the "memory cortex," believing they were stored there. He abandoned this original conclusion in *Mystery of the Mind*, his later book. Sheldrake agrees with Penfield's later position.

Morphic Resonance

Similar things tune into similar systems (Marshall, 1960). Sheldrake posits that we directly tune into the past. You tune into your own past because you are more similar to yourself than someone else. Consider asking a tree, for example, what organism was most similar to this tree in the past? The answer is itself. It is more similar to itself in the past than any other organism.

Self-resonance is the basis of individual memory. We tune into our own past states and enter into a process of morphic resonance with them across time and across space. There is a tuning into our own past and this is how our memory works. This resonance is the same process as to how we tune into a particular thought field, which may incorporate P's.

CHAPTER 15

THE LAWS OF TFT

The benevolence of Natural Law lies in assuring us that...miracles are open to us, but it does not extend to telling us how to accomplish them; it is for us to discover the keys, the encodings and decodings, by which they can be brought to pass.

Robert Rosen
Theoretical Biologist

What are the laws pertaining to psychological problems as uncovered by Thought Field Therapy? This chapter outlines some of these laws. Successful prediction in TFT supports the validity of laws introduced and revealed by the proper application of TFT. As far as I can determine there is no other psychotherapy with the predictive power of Thought Field Therapy.

THE LAW OF THE CORRECT TREATMENTS

The first discovery in TFT was the astonishing fact phobias of all kinds could be cured within minutes. TFT diagnosis revealed that a slightly different and highly specific phobia treatment was required for spiders, claustrophobia, and aircraft turbulence, which was different from the treatment for most of the other phobias. These discoveries were later incorporated into algorithms, simple recipes that almost anyone can follow requiring no special training.

Additional algorithms were developed, through causal diagnosis, for problems such as addiction, depression, anger, jealousy, and obsession. I also discovered by diagnosing individualized TFT treatment sequences, we can eliminate the psychotic-like distortion of body image so common in anorexia. Even paranoid symptoms can be eliminated. However, it was also found that precise, individualized treatments were required for specific problems and, although the nine gamut series and the psychological reversal treatments would help in the treatment of *all* problems, a specific order of the major treatments was found to be required for the rapid differential treatment of varying psychological problems. The accuracy of these requirements is substantiated and borne out in the treatment of more difficult or complex problems with the Voice Technology™ (VT). The VT enables us to help most problems that are unresponsive to our very powerful diagnostic procedures.

Here is a simple example of the importance of order in some cases: A therapist from Italy called me to rave about the wonderful results she was getting in treating food addiction. However, she pointed out, as powerful as the algorithm was for the majority of her clients, she could not get it to work on herself. I said I didn't know why, but got the VT ready and asked her to think of her own hunger. I ran tests on her voice and found that all she needed was a simple change of order, i.e., to put the point first that for most people came second. That was the difference for her—just a simple difference of order in the same major treatment; the nine gamuts remained the same.

The Italian therapist told me she was intensely craving food at that moment, which was why she thought of calling me. When she did the correctly diagnosed, individually prescribed order, her craving immediately and completely disappeared, much to her delight. Usually, in such cases, much more complicated treatments are revealed and necessary for successful treatment. However, in her case, it was merely the simple change of order in how the very same treatments are administered that made the dramatic difference.

Order is as important as it is in opening combination locks. Having merely the numbers in the combination is not sufficient to open the lock; one must put them in the proper order. We find something quite similar in the practice of TFT.

THE LAW OF RAPIDITY

Most experienced psychotherapists have been conditioned to think of rapid therapy as something that can be accomplished in a matter of weeks, hours, or a few months. TFT usually yields dramatic reported treatment effects within minutes—almost instantaneously in many cases! See the Voice Technology™ replication study described in Chapter 5 on Causal Diagnosis. Keep in mind that the people treated had never heard of the procedures before. The reported time measuring the length of therapy *included* explanation of the problem and the necessary instructions of how to do the treatments.

THE LAW OF EFFECTIVENESS OF THERAPY

The tables summarizing the information yielded by the two studies on Voice Technology™ done ten years apart reveal, in addition to the remarkable similarities between the two groups of subjects, the degree of reported effectiveness of the therapy is unprecedented.

THE LAW OF PSYCHOLOGICAL REVERSAL (PR) AND MINI-PSYCHOLOGICAL REVERSAL (MPR)

The laws of PR and MPR are unknown to the client, just as they had been unknown to you. Therefore, it is most interesting to observe the treated naïve client's conformity to these laws. This fact lends greater credence to the reports that they give us, for the reports they give are highly predictable to a knowledgeable TFT therapist in pattern, style and content.

For example, say the client is SUD 10 on a trauma; you administer the first stage of treatment (before the gamut series) and the client reports no change at all—still at a 10. You then correct a psychological reversal and repeat the very same initial procedure before the gamut and the client reports the SUD is now a 7. Since the client does not know about PR nor does he or she understand you were correcting for PR when you did the PR treatment we know the client is likely reporting accurately in reference to changes taking place. The client follows the laws of TFT even though he or she is totally ignorant of what these laws are. The knowledgeable therapist thus has a way of checking on the accuracy of the SUD reports given by clients. We find the reports are almost always very accurate.

When you try to help either yourself or others with the algorithms or recipes provided, you will come upon the extraordinary predictable and lawful phenomenon of psychological reversal and its corollary, mini-psychological reversal, or in sum, the law of reversal. The law of reversal is simply that a person who is in a state (it *is* a state[1]) of reversal is unable to respond to an otherwise effective treatment.

In the case of MPR the same law holds when the person who started at an 8, 9, or 10 on the 10-point scale

---

[1] With our diagnostic procedures, the state of PR or its absence can readily be demonstrated. However, if one has not been trained in these specialized skills, the state is revealed by the phenomenon of non-response to an otherwise effective therapy and then *after* the PR correction is carried out the person responds to the treatment. The PR correction is not in itself a therapy for the problem, but rather opens the path for the therapy to take effect.

gets stuck, say at a 4. We know there was an MPR block-ing the complete effect of the treatment if the person goes to a 1 when the same treatments which a moment before could take the person no lower than a 4 are repeated. In other words, when those same formerly non-effective treat-ments suddenly remove all traces of the problem, then we know there was an MPR blocking the completion of the therapy.

ARCHITECTURE OF TREATMENT AND QUANTUM JUMPS IN THERAPY

As you have learned, TFT provides a particular form, structure or architecture, to therapy. This structure has evolved to include the three main divisions consisting of: 1) what we call the *major treatments* (i.e., the beginning of the eyebrow, eye, arm, collarbone, etc.); 2) the *nine gamut* series of treatments; and 3) the repeat of the very same initial major treatment *sequence* after the nine gamut series has been carried out.

The highly regular pattern of improvement typically and lawfully yields SUD results as follows (assume the cli-ent starts at a 10): 1) after the major treatments the per-son predictably will move from a 10 to the neighborhood of a 7; 2) after the nine gamut series, the person predict-ably will move to about a 4; and then after the repeat of the major sequence the person usually moves to a SUD of 1.

The structure of the treatments was developed through the intensive use of diagnostic procedures over a number of years and revealed the pattern we observe, i.e., majors—nine gamut—repeat of majors. The architecture for typical treatments has been uncovered over a number of years through our diagnostic procedures. The pattern follows the structure: one or more majors—nine gamut treatments—a repeat of the same majors, which were given before the nine gamut treatments. This structure results in improvement that typically shows quantum-type jumps in a predictable common fashion.

The rate of progress, as indicated by the SUD or 10-point scale, will move in distinct quantum-type jumps, without passing through intermediate positions on the SUD scale. This feature is also astonishingly lawful and in all my years of eclectic psychotherapy I never saw or even heard of anything like it. The person who starts with a problem at a 10 for example, will, as therapy progresses, usually in a matter of minutes, move next to 7, then to 4 and then to a 1.

THE LAW OF THE APEX PROBLEM

Perhaps the most surprising lawful, predictable phenomenon revealed in the practice of TFT is what we call the apex problem, called thus when a person is *not* functioning at the apex of his potential mental ability. It consists of the client reporting accurately a dramatic improvement after TFT is carried out but then compulsively attempting to explain away the astonishing results—sometimes "forgetting" there was even a problem—but determinedly avoiding giving credit to the very strange therapy for the improvement. The therapy just seems too peculiar to be able to help a problem.

I treated, over the telephone, a woman with partial paralysis who got extremely frustrated and angry whenever she drops something. She went to a 7 just thinking of dropping an object. After about two minutes of treatment, she paused for quite a while before telling me the after-therapy SUD (an atypical pause on the part of the client is almost a sure sign that an apex is about to be expressed.) When I again asked for the current post-treatment SUD, she said, "Well, it's an underlying thing." She didn't say that prior to the therapy, so I questioned her further and she admitted—and admitted is the correct word—that right now she was unable to get the least bit upset when thinking about dropping things.

CONTROL SYSTEM

The rapid, dramatic and predictable changes accomplished with TFT are evidence that when we do TFT, we are dealing with the control system for negative emotions. When you stand upright, if you pay careful attention, you will observe that you are doing a balancing act and must do this if you are to remain standing. Muscles in your body are operating (now subconsciously, but quite consciously when you were a toddler) automatically to keep you in place; the semi-circular canals in your ear provide continuing information as to your status in space, as does your vision. The feat of standing upright then is due to the operation of a control system. If you are suddenly rendered unconscious you will fall to the ground; the control system for balance is no longer operative. You could also choose to fall down by willfully turning off the control system for balance.

Many people "flew" before the Wright brother's memorable flight. In fact, the Wright brother's flight just before the big success resulted in a bad crash. The brother who piloted the aircraft said with despair after this discouraging crash (echoing their major detractors, including *Scientific American* as well as all the newspapers and most scientists in the country), *"Man will never fly in a thousand years!"* Then they got the brilliant idea of putting a tail-control surface on the plane. This allowed better control. The next flight, only seconds in time and yards in distance, in 1903, was the first *controlled power* flight in aviation history.

The brothers worked purposely with an unstable craft so the pilot could control it. An inherently stable craft is not subject to the same kind of delicate pilot control for which the brothers were aiming. The great breakthrough of control was achieved and soon thereafter gradual, grudging admission of success by others came forth and their work was recognized as a revolutionary breakthrough.

Since TFT practitioners encounter this kind of militant skepticism. For example, *Scientific American*, which would not accept an ad of ours (we wanted to reach some scientists with news of our work), was one of the last to acknowledge the Wright brothers' flight, believing it was *impossible* as most scientists believed at the time. R. Milton's *Alternative Science: Challenging the myths of the scientific establishment* has many relevant facts. The basis of disbelief, which underlies the apex problem, is thoroughly explored in this informative work.

Milton (1996) wrote that the newspapers ignored the brothers, but they began to get pestered, especially the local paper in Dayton where the flights took place:

> In 1940, Dan Kumler, the city editor of the Dayton Daily News at the time of the flights, gave an interview about his refusal to publish anything thirty-five years earlier and spoke frankly about his reasons. Kumler recalled, "We just didn't believe it. Of course, you remember that the Wrights at that time were terribly secretive."

> The interviewer responded incredulously, "You mean they were secretive about the fact that they were flying over an open field?" Kumler considered the question, grinned, and said, "I guess the truth is we were just plain dumb." (p. 12)

> In January, 1906, more than two years after the Wrights had first flown, *Scientific American* carried an article ridiculing the "alleged" flights that the Wrights claimed to have made. Without a trace of irony, the magazine gave as its main reason for not believing the Wrights the fact that the American press had failed to write anything about them." (p.13)

EMOTIONAL CONTROL

In January of 1980, after months or exploration, psychological reversal was discovered. This discovery was soon to be recognized as a crucial contribution to an understanding of the control system for negative emotions, which was soon to be developed. In May of that same

year, Mary, who had been treated by the author unsuc-
cessfully for a year-and-a-half with state of the art conventional therapy methods was instantly cured with an aspect
of the new procedure called Callahan Techniques® to be
later called Thought Field Therapy or simply TFT (Callahan, 1996).

In recognizing the operation of a control system it is
necessary that the observers strive to *see* the evidence in
favor of the system without unjust criticism, which removes
one from the ability to see. The first controlled flight in an
aircraft was only yards in distance and seconds in time.
The results might have been dismissed if the observers
complained: *"Who wants to travel mere yards in an aircraft?"*

Supporting Fact

The fact that an attuned disturbing thought field (i.e.,
one which in our view contains perturbations) can be transformed into a non-disturbing thought field within a matter
of minutes, in a highly predictable fashion, demonstrates
the operation of a control system for the negative emotions (remember, a trained TFT therapist can do this for
almost all psychological problems). The reader of this book
will be able to carry out an experiment to test this on
traumas. The issue of how long this condition will prevail,
though a crucial one for a client and therapist, nevertheless may be seen as irrelevant in terms of evaluating the
function of the control system.

Some years ago, I was suffering from chronic terrible
fatigue and I could find no physician, among dozens tried,
who was able to help me. An acquaintance suggested I

see a particular Chinese acupuncturist, whose family had practiced acupuncture for numerous generations. The gentleman was in his seventies and quite experienced.

In the examination he asked me to describe my complaining symptoms of tiredness and he commented that it was simply a normal symptom of aging. I said I doubted this since there were startling exceptions—there were times when I had enormous energy, and naturally, at such times I was no younger than I was with the fatigue. He did not at all react to this important bit of information, and it appeared that, since it didn't fit his "diagnosis," he chose to ignore it. He put some needles in my arms and legs, and I lay there for a half an hour. When he removed the needles he gave me some herbs, which I was to make into teas and drink. I dutifully followed this advice. Not only did the treatments not help, but the herbs were making me even more fatigued. (I have always been quite dubious of any treatment that is supposed to make you worse before it makes you better. In such cases, I think another treatment ought to be found.)

My main point here is that the exceptions to my fatigue periods proved and demonstrated something of the greatest import. In this case, that my fatigue definitely could not be attributed to my age—I was only in my early fifties and, when not fatigued, looked about ten years younger than my actual age. Years later I found that these exceptional periods of high energy strongly suggested the influence of exogenous factors that I have since identified. Remove the exogenous factors and the fatigue disappears. *The periods of exception designate the potential opera-*

tion of control—even though the periods are relatively brief. Even though one would wish to have high energy at all times, the fact that for short times it is available is revealing of critical and crucial facts.

Voice Technology™ Research

In viewing the data presented in the Causal Diagnosis chapter, it is important not to allow the absence of follow-up data to overwhelm one to the degree that one cannot *see* the data that *is* presented. Actually, no single research study can illustrate everything that might be desired. Our research demonstrates, among other things, that our treatment is far more effective than drugs in eliminating fear. The data illustrate the lawful, predictable, reproducible operation of a control system for the negative emotions. In the history of clinical psychology nothing in any way similar to these data have ever been presented before.

The success reports in causal diagnosis support the existence of a control system for the negative emotions, a control system that responds rapidly and powerfully to the correct and astonishingly minimal input—*when the therapist knows the proper codings.*

As aircraft engineering knowledge developed, the length of time of flight increased. In fact, for the Wright brothers, the length of flight time started increasing dramatically within a short time. In a similar fashion, as TFT has grown and developed over the last twenty years, new discoveries have increased the power of this revolutionary system. In fact, due to the existence of the laws of TFT and the lawful expectation that almost everyone *ought* to be cured of their psychological problems and *remain* cured, it has become possible to make discoveries which have brought those desirable goals ever closer to reality.

How dare I compare TFT to the discovery of the airplane? The airplane, and Young's helicopter, initiated the control of humans in space. TFT initiates an equally exciting period, *the control of inner space*—of ourselves.

THE IMPLICATIONS OF THE LAWS OF TFT

The regularity of the laws revealed by TFT, along with the extraordinary therapy power unveiled, has interesting implications regarding the system responsible for healing. In brief, the evidence suggests that the energy system used in TFT is likely the system of healing used by the body in its homeostatic and natural healing control efforts.

PR for example, as we discussed in the reversal chapter, has been found to be a common characteristic of cancer and many chronic conditions apart from psychological problems. It was found that, upon occasion, merely correcting a PR is sufficient to allow the body to heal an otherwise recalcitrant or chronic problem that had been unresponsive to a number of otherwise potent, effective treatments.

The fact TFT can reproduce certain healing effects that occur naturally lend support to the discovery of a natural control system for the negative emotions. TFT, we believe, is simply tapping into and using the control system which Nature herself uses for healing, growth and maturation.

CHAPTER 16

WHY NIGHTMARES AND OBSESSIONS?

[T]he founder of information theory, Claude Shannon, showed how one could reliably send messages along any channel no matter how noisy: one simply repeats the message again and again. Over the long run the noise averages to zero, while the signal steadily increases. With enough repetition, any signal can be reliably sent through even the noisiest channel.[1]

Mae Won-Ho
Biologist

It is a common experience after terrible events for the victims to have nightmares and/or obsess about the traumatic event. No matter how hard they try,

---

[1] Mae Won-Ho points out Shannon has shown how error can be reduced to any arbitrary desired amount simply by increasing the number of repetitions of the message.

they seem unable to get the experience out of their mind. Everything seems to remind them of it. I believe the nightmares and obsessions were of enormous value from an evolutionary survival standpoint. In order to understand this it is necessary to know something of the brilliant biological theory put forth by biologist Rupert Sheldrake.[2]

I believe traumatic episodes are repeated through obsession and nightmares so the information related to the events, along with intense and appropriate emotional upset (perturbations) can be accurately transmitted to future generations for their potential protection, safety and survival. One might think this information could only be transmitted to future generations through genetic means, but this is precisely what Sheldrake (1989) challenges. He offers what I believe (and my work supports) is a more comprehensive solution.

Our work conclusively proves that memory of the traumatic event is not the problem in trauma since after our trauma treatment the person remembers details of the event as well as, or usually even better than prior to the treatment. However, after treatment, the memory is no longer loaded with upset, and the nightmares and the obsession over the event are gone. This robust and easily reproducible fact is the main reason why I was forced to come up with a radical new theory[3] as to why trauma victims suffer from obsession and nightmares about the trauma.

---

[2] Sheldrake's ideas are available at http://www.sheldrake.org

[3] I have heard professionals call this a "repetition compulsion," but this is a *description,* not an explanation.

A trauma creates a perturbation in a thought field. The perturbation (P), rather than the trauma itself, is what is responsible for nightmares and for obsession, as well as the intense emotional upset. The evidence for this is our treatment—when we eliminate the P's with TFT, the emotional upset as well as the nightmares and the obsessions are gone. This is a blessing of nature, for if it were the trauma itself, no help would be available. Thought Field Therapy collapses the P and the disturbance is gone. TFT eliminates the perturbations, which are *not the upset* but rather are the deepest and most fundamental *cause* of emotional upset. After successful trauma treatment, then the victim is free to remember all the horrible details of the event without getting upset.

WHY NIGHTMARES AND OBSESSIONS?

Since TFT is so effective in eliminating the upset following a trauma, including the complicating sequelae of nightmares and obsessions, I wondered what purpose was being served by such symptoms? I believe nightmares and obsessions about the traumatic event have served a vital life-preserving function.

To preserve and protect life, it is important to know something about the nature of the dangers that can threaten life in order to avoid or minimize such dangers. For example, all land-based chordates develop, as soon as self-initiated movement begins,[4] a fear of heights. Ants

---

[4] One is unable to *perceive* a declivity or a height unless self-initiated movement has taken place (Gibson, 1962).

and fish, for example, have no need for such a fear and hence show no trace of it.

Information about the danger of heights obviously had to be learned at some point in the past. The way this was initially learned was through traumas resulting from falling and through witnessing others of the same species, perhaps even family members, become hurt through actual falls. The upset, obsessions and nightmares that stemmed from these traumas would put information into the collective unconscious, or collective field.

WITNESSING TRAUMA IS ITSELF TRAUMATIC

Witnessing a trauma is itself traumatic and may lead to obsession and nightmares. Dr. Freinkel, a psychiatrist at Stanford University School of Medicine, and his co-workers reported a study on journalists who experienced executions. Even though the executions were legal, many of the reporters witnessing these sanctioned killings experienced symptoms of trauma. Dr. Freinkel (1994) said: "For the first time...evidence suggests that merely witnessing violence—even if the act has legal approval and observers prepare for it in advance—provides at least short-lived dissociation and anxiety."

Witnesses to trauma who experience traumatic symptoms themselves contribute additional information input to the collective data bank. If one is killed in a traumatic situation, there can be no obsessions or nightmares, and hence no information emanating from the individuals who are killed.[5] Having witnesses helps send vital information out to future individuals by way of the collective unconscious.

To understand more specifically the reason for the symptoms of obsession and nightmares in response to traumas, it is necessary first to know something about a brilliant biological theory put forth by the British scientist Rupert Sheldrake (1987, 1989). Among many other things, his theory can explain some issues that are not well explained in conventional biology, such as how is the information in instincts transmitted? I cannot do justice to Dr. Sheldrake's work here and I strongly recommend the interested reader study the two books which present his theory—*A New Science of Life* and *The Presence of the Past.* First we must consider instinct.

WHAT IS INSTINCT?

"Instinct can be...regarded as a fixed pattern of activity inherited by the species collectively from behavior learned earlier in its history." (Young, 1979b, p. 155). This concise, simple and accurate statement led me to look up Arthur M. Young, inventor of the Bell helicopter, and study his works.

At one time in ancient history all of the information that is now contained in instincts had to be learned. If it had to be learned afresh in each generation, life might not have survived. But the information clearly pertains to this world and could only be learned in this world. But hard-

---

[5] Since almost all bulls are killed in bullfights, this explains why they do not attempt to run out of the ring as soon as they enter it.

won knowledge can be passed on to future generations; the question is how? Sheldrake provides the most satisfactory answer to this question that I have come across. We explain such puzzling things as bird navigation by calling them instinct. If anyone has taken training in celestial navigation, one can appreciate the amount of knowledge and information that must be contained in this instinct which allows birds to navigate accurately over long distances.

There are many astonishing examples of what we call instinct and here are two I find challenging from a theoretical perspective: Prior to laying its eggs, the tarantula hawk wasp selects a tarantula and then does some very careful and precise neurological surgery. It stings the tarantula in the exact spot that results in paralysis but not death. This delicate surgical procedure ensures the future young of the wasp will have fresh food to feed upon while they are developing.

The nests birds build represent a vast amount of detailed information on the selection of building materials, as well as complex structural engineering. This information is adapted to radically varying conditions and circumstances. We tend to take bird nests for granted since they are so commonplace. However, there is an interesting one-celled animal called Foraminifera, which lives on the

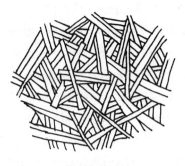

ocean floor. This one celled animal—with no known nervous system[6] and no brain—selects spicules, which are small pieces of sponges from the ocean floor and weaves these especially selected spicules into an elaborate and close-fitting microscopic-size nest. Some biologists inform us that the information required to perform such exquisitely refined behavior is in the genes. The evidence of my work forced me to abandon this idea.

Some scientists are satisfied to explain the amazing creativity involved in building such a thing as an elaborate nest by calling it instinct. But instinct means it is done automatically, such as when we drive a car or play the piano and we don't have to think about it anymore since it is so well practiced. But there had to be a first time—such intricate phenomena do not just pop up by acci-

---

[6] Every living cell is composed of microtubules. Stuart Hameroff (an anesthesiologist) and Roger Penrose (a brilliant mathematical physicist who was Stephen Hawking's professor), in their creative efforts to understand the puzzling phenomenon of consciousness have put forth an elaborate theory involving these microtubules that is most interesting. It seems a distinct possibility that the microtubules may serve as a "nervous" or communication system in such animals and perhaps in all animals. See drawing of elaborate nest made by Foraminifera, a one-celled animal.

dent. An individual Foraminiferum had to first come up with this solution. Perhaps others later modified and worked with the nest idea but one had to be the first.

The cover article of *Science News* by Susan Milius (June 5, 1999) reports on scientists who have been studying creativity in animals such as guppies, birds, and other animals. Sheldrake (1989) reports extensively on the creativity of the blue tit birds that opened milk bottles to get the cream off the top. Milius reports on the chickadees that learned how to open the coffee cream containers that restaurants use. Milius reports a house sparrow hovering in front of the sensor that triggers the automatic door at a bus stop and then flying inside for food.

I have been observing flies for years and noted how cleverly some will stay out of sight of the screen or solid door until the door opens and then they zoom in the house as if coming out of nowhere, before it is possible to close the door. This is intelligent and creative behavior.

Chimps clearly invent things, reports Sarah T. Boysen, who runs the primate lab at Ohio State. "I see something just about every day." (Milius, p. 365)

Discovery Always by an Individual

It has been known for years human discovery is always by an individual and interestingly the same is being found with animals. Boysen points out classic evolutionary theory "emphasized population processes but to appreciate innovation, the individual becomes very important."

In a comment that human radical innovators can easily agree with, Boysen speculates part of this reason may lie in the very low status of innovators: the poor competitors, the small, and the hungry—and I would add, "the odd balls." Also, I might say, the more the radical innovations become known, the lower the status becomes.

As Machiavelli observed in *The Prince*: "There is nothing more difficult to take in hand, more perilous to conduct, or more uncertain in its success, than to take the lead in the introduction of a new order of things, because the innovator has for enemies all those who have done well under the old conditions, and lukewarm defenders in those who may do well under the new."

No Genetic Engineering Required

Having been well trained in evolution and heredity, I knew phobias were largely inherited. Rarely is a phobia due to a past trauma experienced by that individual (see Hugdahl and Kiarker, 1981, and Seligman, 1941). However, it is my thesis that inherited phobias (which the include the majority) are due to the collected traumas of eons ago. The first fact that caused me to question the validity that genes (DNA) contained the elaborate inherited psychological information as commonly represented in instincts or fears and phobias, is the robust ease with which I was able to cure phobias with my new discovery (Callahan, 1985 and 1993a).

If the cause of the phobia were hard-wired somehow in the genes or even in the brain, then my simple treatments *should not be able to eliminate these problems.* I am doing no brain surgery, adding no foreign chemicals to the person (though I am obviously changing the body chemistry in a natural way). I am certainly not doing genetic engineering in my simple but powerful treatments. Yet, the highly ordered information-generating severe emotional distress evident in phobias is rendered neutral or gone due to the simple, *non-invasive, natural* treatments I apply.

In my undergraduate days at the University of Michigan, I was fortunate to have as a professor, A. Franklin Shull, who was an expert on genetics and evolution. Due to the influence of his courses, I have had a continuing appreciation of the role of heredity in psychological problems. Until recently, I assumed heredity must necessarily mean genetics, or DNA-determined, but I no longer believe that.

Conventional theory teaches us all the information evident in instincts must, and can only, come from the DNA in the genes. It is well established that the genes do govern the formulation of the physical materials in the development of living entities, but anything beyond this is speculative. The elaborate information contained in instincts supposedly being in the DNA I believe is an error.

Paul Davies (1988), an astrophysicist, puts the problem very succinctly: "But in the absence of an explanation for how an arrangement of molecules (DNA) translate into a behavioral skill that can accommodate completely unforeseen disruptions (such as entailed in bird navigation) this is little more than hand-waving. When it comes to animal behavior, the relevant concepts are information in character." (p. 188) Davies says the genetic theory implies that the DNA (a chemical molecule) could somehow yield a map displaying where all the stars are in celestial navigation by birds. The current genetic theory explaining instincts creates more problems than it solves.

Sheldrake maintains that the idea of DNA shaping the organism or programming its behavior is a quite illegitimate extrapolation from anything we know about what DNA does. What we know is that DNA codes the sequence of the amino acids in proteins and plays a role in the control of the synthesis of protein. Sheldrake suggests all of the unsolved problems in biology are being attributed to DNA. He proposes that DNA has been turned into a kind of mystical theory in which DNA is used to explain almost everything.

Nobel Laureate Brian Goodwin (1988), in his review of a book by Ian Stewart, states: "In this [book] you also get important insights into biology from someone who sees the subject in a refreshingly different light from the narrow beams of the dominant gang of genetic reductionists." Goodwin concludes his review by speculating why biologists cling to genes and information: "Maybe it's the lack of mathematics and physics in biological education that biases evolutionary thinking towards genes and information." Life's other secret is order. In the hierarchy of life, order is all-important. Goodwin adds: "The key is in spotting the order, which can be very subtle."[7]

---

[7] Discovering the order in disorders is a shorthand way to characterize my discoveries.

A Resonance Theory of Memory

In 1960, Ninian Marshall proposed a very interesting physical theory of memory, which also would provide a scientific explanation for ESP. Sheldrake credits Marshall's work for helping him to think about the much more detailed biological theory of morphic resonance.

Marshall states, "Telepathy...is the partial reproduction in one brain of a pattern in another brain." (p. 266) Interestingly, since the time this seemingly radical notion was proposed, there has been a recent experiment which lends strong experimental support to the actual possibility of this idea (see Grinberg-Zylerbaum, 1992, 1997, 1998, 1992). A description of this latter experiment is described in Goswami (1993, 132-3).

Organ Transplants

In every organ in the body, in every cell—all of the atoms are vibrating. The rate of vibration is what sets the stage for resonance tuning. It is commonly reported that people who receive organ transplants appear to have some of the memories and tastes of the donor. Claire Sylvia received the heart and lungs of a young man killed in an accident. She found herself having unusual cravings. She had never cared for beer, but after the transplant she craved beer and also suddenly discovered other unusual (for her) tastes.

Paul Pearsall (1998) reports on a number of organ transplant patients and tells of an eight-year-old girl who received the heart of a murdered ten-year-old girl. The recipient began having nightmares about the other girl's murderer and was reportedly able to provide a detailed description of the man in sufficient detail to allow the police to track down and convict the murderer. Pearsall also tells of a middle-aged man whose taste in music was radically altered when he received the heart of a teenager.

Scientists feel uncomfortable with such reports because they have no explanation for such things. However, these reports can readily be explained by Sheldrake's theory of morphic resonance.

Faster-than-Light Communication?

In physics an unusual phenomenon involving a strange interconnection between atomic particles is called the Einstein-Podolsky-Rosen (EPR) effect. Their article was published in 1935. It is ironic this group of eminent physicists was attempting to show an absurdity and incompleteness in quantum theory in their article. They pointed out quantum theory would predict that if two particles were once connected and then separated, even by light years, a change in one of the particles would immediately demand an opposite change in the other particle. This would violate Einstein's dictum nothing can travel faster than light. For years this "absurdity" could only remain a serious speculation in quantum theory.

Irish physicist John Bell (1965) developed a thought experiment, which would decide, once and for all, for or against quantum physics and this strange, supposed interconnection. Inspired by David Bohm's work on non-local "hidden variables" proposed for quantum theory, Bell came up with an experimental solution to the EPR position (Fry, 1993, p. 54). Fry states, "The remarkable Einstein-Podolsky-Rosen correlations (Aspect, Bell) have defied any reasonable classical kind of explanation." (p. 542) Which indicates that EPR was mistaken, according to now overwhelming cumulative evidence. Henry Stapp (1977), theoretical physicist, says, "Bell's Theorem is the most profound discovery in science."

Years later, French physicist Alain Aspect and his colleagues actually carried out a crucial experiment that stunningly substantiated the strange prediction from quantum theory. The experiment has now been done a number of times with various refinements so physicists now accept quantum theory is correct and Einstein was mistaken. As odd as it seems, two particles once connected appear to maintain a strange connection over great distances, in space and time, even though light years apart.

Non-Locality and Brain Resonance

As suggested by Marshall (above), Goswami believes the EPR phenomenon may have an equivalent counterpart in consciousness or specifically in brains. A most interesting experiment is reported in Goswami (1993):

> A recent experiment by the Mexican neurophysiologist Jacobo Grinberg-Zylberbaum and his collaborators directly supports the idea of nonlocality in human brain-minds—this experiment is the brain equivalent of Aspect's (photon) experiment. Two subjects are instructed to interact for a period of thirty or forty minutes until they start feeling a "direct communication." They then enter separate Fara-

day cages (metallic enclosures that block all electromagnetic signals). Unbeknownst to his or her partner, one of the subjects is now shown a flickering light signal that produces an evoked potential (an electrophysiological response produced by a sensory stimulus and measured by an EEG) in the light-stimulated brain. But amazingly, as long as the partners in the experiment maintain their direct communication, the unstimulated brain also shows an electrophysiological activity, called a transfer potential, quite similar in shape and strength to the evoked potential of the stimulated brain. (In contrast, control subject does not show a transfer potential.) The straightforward explanation is quantum nonlocality: The two brain-minds act as a nonlocally correlated system—the correlations established and maintained through nonlocal consciousness—by virtue of the quantum nature of the brains. (p. 132)

None of the subjects reported any conscious awareness of the transfer potential. The results were only clear when the correlation of the two potentials were compared. Goswami says, "This is similar to the situation in Aspect's experiment."

MORPHIC RESONANCE AND THE COLLECTIVE UNCONSCIOUS

Sheldrake has proposed a most interesting theory, which he calls Morphic Resonance. When you tune your radio or your television set, you are adjusting the circuitry so that it is in resonance with a particular transmitter. You change the tuning circuit somewhat and you can receive a different station.

In the realm of behavior, self-resonance is the basis of individual memory (Sheldrake, Ninian Marshall). We tune into our own past states and enter into a process of morphic resonance with them across time and across space. There is a tuning into our own past. This is how our memory works. This resonance is basically how we tune into a thought field, which may incorporate perturbations.

When I first heard of Carl Jung's notion of a collective unconscious as a graduate student, I rejected it out of hand as being impossible. However, the development of my discoveries has obliged me to radically reassess this notion. I am now convinced there is a collective unconscious and, among other things, it can account for complex instinctual information being passed on to future generations.

Sheldrake's theory of morphic resonance gives a theoretical scientific explanation for a means by which the collective unconscious could become established. It is also able to answer the issue of instincts and how they may be passed on. We tune into a memory of habits—we do not get flashes of millions of people's previous experiences— we get a kind of average of these impressions. Archetypal or average or probable patterns are attuned based upon input of all members of a particular group. There is a collective quality to these memories. Essentially archetypal behavior or thoughts and experiences are the material that is tuned.

There is a certain similarity here to the idea of Jung (1953), a collective memory that is unconscious. Jung showed striking similarities between dreams of people in one part of the world with myths in other parts. The idea ran into trouble with mechanistic biologists who believe there is no known mechanism or way for such to happen. In the current conventional approach there is no way the myths of one tribe on the other part of the world could get into the dreams of people in Switzerland.

The collective unconscious made no sense in conventional terms. This is the main reason the collective unconscious has never been accepted in biology. But it, or something like it, seems necessary to explain certain facts such as instinct. We know electromagnetic radiation can carry vast information such as that received by radio and television receivers. Something quite different but perhaps with a certain similarity to EMG radiation may well be involved.

Sheldrake states that to assume memories and programs are in the brain would be analogous to assuming that TV programs and radio programs were somehow within the sets. I remember clearly having a similar theory to the current brain theory when I was a young child. I recall being intrigued with the music being sung by people, and I assumed these people must somehow be inside the old fashioned wind-up record player (Victrola). I used to explore, as best I could, within the cabinet hoping to catch sight of what had to be extremely little people. Being Irish, I had heard of the little people and hoped to catch a glimpse before they could hide. I never did. I now understand that waves of compressed information were impressed upon the solid records.

Actually what is in radio and TV sets, among other things, are tuning circuits, which bring in a particular program when the resonance of the circuits in the set is tuned to match the resonance of a particular transmitter. The resonance model seems a much more reasonable one than the notion that everything is in the brain.

SUMMARY

Why do people (and animals) have nightmares and obsess about traumas? I propose that this is the means nature has devised for getting accurate information to future creatures regarding potential dangers in the world. Claude Shannon (1949) has shown the value of repeating messages in a noisy channel. When one considers all the thoughts, all the emotions that are collectively going on at any one time, the channels are quite full of noise. In order to get vital potential life-saving information into the channels it must be repeated over and over again.

The more trauma victims or witnesses obsess about a trauma and the more nightmares they have pertaining to the trauma, the more clear the messages regarding the real dangers in the world. Do we need this? Humans have developed elaborate means of education and passing on information (e.g., books, letters, newspapers, radio, and television). We humans no longer need to suffer the problems of obsession and nightmares in order to get information out regarding dangers in the world in order to protect our offspring. Our problems for the future lie in a completely different domain, and that is how to prevent nuclear war and other destructive derivatives of scientific progress.

All phobias are due to trauma, but not in the current lifetime but rather traumas collectively accumulated from the ancient past. Although Shannon discovered the laws fundamental to information theory, Loewenstein (1999, p. 184) points out that evolution has been using these principles for eons. Nature has created and also has been using for eons the intricate and brilliant control system for healing, which is now available for the benefit of all.

CHAPTER 17

NATURAL TREATMENT

If you have looked at the treatment presented here and examined the data reported in Chapter 5, Causal Diagnosis, it should be clear that TFT treatment is a simple, effective, and non-invasive procedure. The treatments are gentle, and use the body's natural control system. The treatment releases the powerful and natural tendency toward healing which is present in all healthy living creatures. The evidence from this treatment suggests that this marvelous healing power within is just waiting for the correct taps to release it and set it free.

I was surprised to discover that the trauma treatment worked so effectively when I first discovered it. Why? Because the upset as a result of trauma is normal and warranted. I was surprised that normal, intense upsetting emotions could be eliminated with such incredible ease. With psychological problems such as unwarranted depression, anxiety, or fears, it seems more reasonable we could

put a person back into balance and eliminate the seeming unjustifiable emotion.

Following two decades of experience using this treatment, with thousands of people all over the world, we
know with confidence that the treatment either helps or it
does nothing. It is non-invasive and does no harm. The
procedure is brief, yet powerful. There has never been a
treatment to relieve and cure a psychological problem
with the power of Thought Field Therapy when it is properly done.

It is important to understand there are other psychological treatments that re-traumatize the victim. In fact,
there are some "treatments" that intentionally upset and
bother the person. Therapists who use such methods believe, quite mistakenly in my view, this will prove helpful.
I compare such treatments to the very old-fashioned medical treatment of bloodletting.

DRUGS

Those of us who use these natural treatments find
they are far more powerful than drugs and, unlike drugs
and some other psychological treatments, have no harmful side effects.

Drugs are a multi-billion-dollar industry. Most people
have been conditioned to go to their doctor and get a pill
to help their problem. The problem with using drugs to
treat psychological problems is three-fold:

1. The drugs, as mentioned are not as effective as
   this therapy.

2. The drugs have side-effects and can cause serious harm, especially when used over time.

3. Drugs are not curative, but must continually be used to gain some measure of relief. Such relief is gained by masking awareness to some degree and therefore normal activities such as driving or working may be impaired.

Many people are not aware of the alarming fact that at least 140,000 people are killed every year in the U.S. due to prescribed medications. This is a particular problem with the elderly who, as a group, face or have faced a higher a number of traumatic events such as the death of loved ones, terminal illness, injuries, life-threatening and chronic illness, etc.

Tragically, many physicians today receive most of their information about drugs from drug salesmen. Drug companies pour vast sums of money into medical activities, professional medical meetings and entertainment of the profession. Fortunately, today there is a major increase in consumer awareness and a strong trend toward what is called alternative, or holistic, approaches in medicine. These terms usually refer to less risky interventions like homeopathy, naturopathy, chiropractic and acupuncture. More and more traditionally trained physicians are exploring less harmful methods of helping people.

In psychology there is an opposite trend. There is a movement to obtain prescription privileges for specially trained post-doctoral psychologists. Special courses and examinations, as well as years of post-doctoral study, are required for a psychologist to achieve a diploma in this specialty. These highly qualified professionals are waiting only for appropriate laws to be passed that will allow them to prescribe drugs.

Back in the middle 1950s, I was a research clinical psychologist and along with a Professor of Pediatrics at the University of Michigan, Dr. B. Graham, and another psychologist Dr. Sydney Rosenblum, carried out the first double-blind study ever performed on psychotropic medication. We were very excited about the possibilities of these medications to help our patient population. Alas, much to our surprise, we found no supporting evidence for the use of these medications with this disturbed population. This study (Graham, 1958) was published in *The Journal of Diseases of Children*. The major drug company that funded this study and provided the medications and the placebos (a pill disguised to look like the drug), naturally did not give us any further funds for research.

PROPER NUTRITION CAN HELP

Many people are more vulnerable to psychological and other health problems because they do not receive proper nutrition. Personally, I have been very interested in nutrition for about forty years. Years ago, I was a member of two organizations devoted to proper nutrition and health. Linus Pauling, who won two Nobel Prizes, one for chemistry and one for peace, was the originator and source of inspiration for these organizations. They were, Orthomolecular Medicine and Orthomolecular Psychiatry. In fact, the president of Orthomolecular Psychiatry at the time was Harvey Ross, MD, who first introduced me to a procedure derived from Applied Kinesiology. This was the beginning of the development of the Callahan Techniques® and Thought Field Therapy.

Dr. Earl Mindell has been a pioneer in nutrition for health for thirty years. His book *Earl Mindell's Vitamin Bible for the 21st Century*[1] is known throughout the world and has sold over nine million copies. In recent years he has been formulating an exclusive line of nutritional products. Over the years, I have used a number of the top nutritional lines and personally have benefited more from Dr. Mindell's formulations than any of the others. Dr. Mindell has the ambitious goal of emptying the hospitals of the many people who are there simply because they do not have adequate nutritional intake or are unnecessarily over-medicated. Dr. Mindell has another book of central interest to psychologists and psychotherapists titled *The Prescription Alternative*. This book provides natural and healthy alternatives to common and popular prescribed drugs.

No Further Interest in Prescribing Drugs

Two of my trainees in Voice Technology™ are diplomates in the specialty of prescribing medications. They are Stephen Daniel, Ph.D., FPPR,[2] VT, and Gale Joslin, Ph.D., FPPR, VT. Each of these highly qualified psycholo-

---

[1] This is the title of the latest revised edition.
[2] The letters FPPR indicate that one is a fellow of the Prescribing Psychologists' Register. This designation shows one is a board-certified diplomate fellow of that organization which represents years of postgraduate study in that specialty.

gists say that if he had learned TFT Voice Technology™ prior to taking the involved courses of study leading to their diplomate in prescribing, they would not have bothered. Why? Because these psychotherapists have found they can get better results with TFT and without the risk of side effects to their clients. Recently, at my request, they sent me the following e-mail letters which I am reprinting with their permission.

Subject: Re: drugs

Roger.

The letters FPPR stand for fellow-diplomate in psychopharmacology from the prescribing psychologist register. What it means is that I have enough knowledge after a 4-year post doc in psychopharmacology, that there is NO WAY I would ever prescribe even if I had the legal ability to do so.

In the last course, a psychiatrist described this case:

A 22-year-old bulimic, bipolar was put on valproic acid, she immediately lost all the hair on her body. They next put her on lithium, where she developed severe face-scarring acne, and gained 52 lbs. Next they put her on tegretol, where she developed orthostatic hypotension, got dizzy and fell down a flight of stairs, breaking her ankle. The question was what would I do?

My answer: TFT Voice Technology™, of course. The new standard, according to the psychiatrist who is also an attorney, is that the doctor has to explain all possible medication interactions and side effects, and MUST INFORM THE PATIENT OF ANY HOLISTIC ALTERNATIVES TO THE MEDICATION HE IS RECOMMENDING. I can't image any patient wanting drugs after I have given the data on any drug vs. TFT.

Stephen Daniel

P.S. The above came out of an ethics lecture by a psychiatrist who is also an attorney at law. He presented at the Prescribing Psychologist Register lecture series #17 in Las Vegas Nevada. The patient mentioned was not his, nor did he present the case, it was presented by another psychiatrist.

I can just imagine an attorney in a court case where I had prescribed drugs. He or she would say: "Dr. Daniel, given the phenomenal success of TFT-VT from your own research, and the fact it has never harmed anyone, WHY THE HELL DID YOU GIVE MY CLIENT THESE TOXIC DRUGS THAT CAUSED MEMORY LOSS, LOSS OF SEXUAL FUNCTION, WEIGHT GAIN, HEART TOXICITY, BOWEL OBSTRUCTION, HAIR LOSS, TRIGGERED A MANIC PHASE, NAUSEA, TARDIVE DYSKENSIA, TREMORS, ORTHOSTATIC HYPOTENSION...ETC.?

Roger, you can see how I could never give drugs with the knowledge I have of TFT. Furthermore, if I explained to the client all the possible drug effects, the success rate of drugs, and then the effectiveness of TFT and its lack of side effects; and if at that point the client chose drugs over TFT, any attorney could make a good case that they were out of their mind at that point, and unable to function mentally well enough to give legal consent!

Stephen Daniel

Here is a letter from another VT-trained psychologist: He started his psychopharmacology training in 1995:

I just recently finished my last class after four years, and I will take the national exam in September 1999. After that, I will be one of 500 psychologists in the United States who is qualified to prescribe medication. All that is needed after that is state-by-state approval. That will be forthcoming as Guam, a United States Territory, allows psychologists to prescribe now.

Having said all this, if I had known of TFT, and especially VT, I would not have taken prescription training. The things I can sometimes do with VT are impossible with medication. Many patients come to me after they have been on medication for VT help with their problem.

One of the good things about having the knowledge to prescribe is you don't have to prescribe.

Many of the antidepressants and anti-anxiety drugs have major side effects. Why give someone drugs when you can do VT, which has NO side effects? Or as one of my patients, who has experienced VT, says VT has no side effects unless you consider positive side effects of good mental outlook and a happy, healthy life.

There are some patients who are not receptive to doing VT; they would prefer medication. However, many of them try VT after the medication doesn't perform as they had hoped. Then they typically say, "they should have done VT first." If given a choice, I will use TFT VT with patients before I try medication. With VT, I can offer my patients a more well rounded approach to their problems; one where we use the body's natural mechanisms, one where the patient has complete control over their own life.

Gale Joslin

CHAPTER 18

TFT AND HEART RATE VARIABILITY

The HRV can be used as a simple tool for monitoring therapeutic effectiveness.

Donald Singer and Zsolt Ori

The Heart Rate Variability test...gives an incredibly accurate view of the autonomic nervous system as well as the variability of the heart. What I found is that TFT, which I have been using, has a dramatic effect on the autonomic nervous system (ANS) in correcting disorders involved in the parasympathetic and sympathetic nervous system.... It is extremely difficult to change the ANS because it is a stable characteristic. There is no placebo effect with the ANS.... TFT has been for me a nice piece of the puzzle that's been missing as to how to enter and

231

correct rapidly defects in the autonomic nervous system.

Fuller Royal, MD
Medical Director, The Nevada Clinic

I t is well known that various emotional problems can contribute to increased risk for individuals with heart difficulties. In some cases, the emotional problems may influence the development of a heart or other organ difficulty. It has been well documented that anger and rage are hazardous to the heart and it is also commonly observed that depression contributes to early death after a heart problem.

HEART RATE VARIABILITY (HRV)

At one time it was believed that the rhythm of the heartbeat should be perfectly even. However, in 1965, Hon and Lee noted that fetal distress was associated with "alterations in interbeat intervals before any appreciable change occurred in heart rate itself." In 1996, Sayers and others focused attention on the existence of physiological rhythms imbedded in the beat-to-beat heart rate signal. (Task Force, 1996, p. 1043)

Although the procedure to measure the variation in the intervals between heartbeats is called *heart rate variability* (HRV) it is not the heart rate itself that is being addressed, but rather the intervals between heart beats. Research found that an even interval is a danger signal and a predictor of mortality. What is desired is a form of chaos, which appears to be associated with information processing and health. The software involved in HRV is complex and derived from physics and electrophysiology. "Rhythmicity, a major feature of the electrocardiogram (ECG) signal, is a characteristic of biological systems and deviations from rhythmicity are often associated with information transfer." (Schmidt and Morfill, p. 87)

A new and exciting field in cardiologic research is developing through the use of instruments that measure HRV. The HRV instrument yields a number of important indices and has become a marker for, among other things, the degree of balance or imbalance in the autonomic nervous system. (Malik and Malik and Camm)

HRV results are stable and unresponsive to placebo. "HRV parameters were studied in order to assess their reproducibility between baseline and placebo (i.e., when receiving placebo therapy.... Surprisingly, the mean and standard deviations of all HRV measures were identical between placebo and baseline measurements...." (Kautzner, p. 167). A similar position is reinforced (Bosner and Kleiger, 1995, p. 338) by other authors: "[T]he lack of placebo effect and the limited individual variability in their measurement made them suitable variables for the study of interventions on autonomic tone." They point out this has been verified by P.E. Stein in an unpublished study. *These factors make HRV a desirable objective physiological measure to evaluate therapy.*

How I Was Introduced to HRV

In July 1997 I received a phone call from Fuller Royal, MD, chief of a medical clinic in Las Vegas. He told me of some astonishing findings while experimenting with one of my simple algorithms for phobias in treating medical patients and measuring the results with the cardiology procedure called heart rate variability. It makes sense that the phobia algorithm might help HRV when one views the results of Kawachi, et al. (1995). They found people with phobias had lower heart variability scores and therefore would be more prone to heart problems.

To my great surprise, I witnessed Dr. Royal proceed to eliminate *all traces of medical symptoms* in twelve patients using my simple algorithm. These dramatic results were then validated by HRV, which showed dramatic improvements for each. (This is documented in our TFT and HRV video.) Interestingly, the patients responded in our time-tested fashion, i.e., they progressed as the algorithm progressed. When the patient did not respond, Dr. Royal would do the PR correction and repeat the algorithm. The patient would then, predictably, respond favorably.

The variability in the heart rate is being used as an objective measure of what is happening, among other things, in the autonomic nervous system. Interest in HRV is growing and in the near future, most physicians, and especially most psychotherapists, will doubtless have this equipment in their offices since it will give them immediate, objective feedback and evidence as to the power of various treatments they are administering.

In my opinion, within the near future all psychotherapies will necessarily be tested with this objective measure. This objective instrument is known to be free of placebo influence and, as more psychotherapists begin to use HRV, we will see an end to testing psychotherapies with a control group and statistical tests in the attempt to demonstrate that the miniscule effects of most feeble conventional approaches are greater than chance.

It is important to understand that when we measure the HRV, the client is tuned to his most severe problem. After TFT treatment, the person again thinks of the same problem and we see profound physiological differences immediately, due to the treatment. Some professionals who use HRV attempt to get the person to think warm and loving thoughts in order to be distracted from their problems. We do a quite different procedure. We ask the person to think of their most disturbing thought and then we remove all discomfort associated with that thought. In this way we are removing the cause (perturbations) of the problem. After TFT treatment the most disturbing thought loses all power to cause upset. The HRV then shows dramatic physiologic changes corresponding to the client's report of dramatic psychological changes.

The HRV started as a clinical and research tool for cardiologists, but its influence in clinical psychology, psychiatry, and general medicine is growing rapidly. More and more investigators are using HRV in the domain of psychological problems. See the applications by Carney et al; Friedman, B.H. and Thayer, J.F. (1998a); Friedman, B.H., and Thayer, F.J., (1998b); Kawachi; Komatusu T., Kimura T., Sanchala V., et al. (1995); Langewitz W., and Ruddel H.; Lehofer, M., et al; McCraty, R., et al; Malik and Camm (1995); and Yeragani, V.K., et al. (1991, 1998).

HRV EXPERTS SURPRISED BY TFT IMPACT

Recently, Ian Graham of the United Kingdom, reported on the first International TFT Conference in Oslo, Norway. Ian reports (Graham, 1999):

> John Hetlelid, a Norwegian expert in the field of Heart Rate Variability testing was next to speak. He expressed his own astonishment at the instantaneous impact of TFT on HRV—apparently on testing TFT for the first time he was convinced that there was an error in the data he obtained. Only when the test was repeated with the same result did he believe what he had witnessed! Much data was then presented that confirmed TFT's capability. He is now analyzing TFT treatment point by treatment point, to determine the relative contribution of each to successful treatment.[1]

It has become commonplace to get such reactions from professionals who are experts in HRV. Many of these experts then explore the rapid effects of TFT and become excited about TFT as a treatment with great potential to improve the HRV results.

---

[1] My prediction on this matter is that the last one in an effective series will show as effective even though the preceding points may have been required, just as in a combination lock. One might get the impression that only the last number is relevant in a combination lock but the last would have not been able to do the job unless the preceding numbers were entered in the correct order. Also, there will be individual variation as in all human matters.

CASE STUDY IN HRV AND CAUSAL DIAGNOSIS

Since Dr. Fuller Royal's discovery of the power of TFT on improving measures of HRV (Callahan, 1997), I felt it was worthwhile to see if my work could help heart problems for patients under the care of a cardiologist. The day after I viewed Dr. Royal's HRV results using TFT, I received a call from a person I will call "Jim," who was in a hospital's intensive care unit (ICU). He was not calling for help but perhaps calling to say "goodbye" in case he did not survive the severe attack he was having of atrial fibrillation. The drugs were not helping and, in fact, it was found later, he had been given one drug to which he was found to be severely allergic. This drug was worsening his condition.

If it were not for my experience at Dr. Royal's clinic, it never would have entered my mind to even attempt to help such a problem as atrial fibrillation. I readied the Voice Technology™ (VT) and led Jim through a number of treatments. It took about fifteen minutes. Despite the toxic chemical opposition of the drug, the treatments were able to do the job. About a half-hour later, Jim called back and said the atrial fibrillation had stopped! This was in July 1997. Two years later, Jim was in town and I had some HRV measuring equipment handy. I wanted to see how he would show up on this diagnostic equipment, which I had not had earlier. I took an HRV reading prior to treatment. Then I had him do an algorithm and took another reading. Then I treated him with Voice Technology™ and did still another reading. Here is a brief summary of the results (interested professionals can get copies of the complete results by contacting me). These results clearly show the progressive power of our treatments as one goes from algorithm to VT.

The following scores are from a program called Freeze-Framer™, which is useful but does not give the range of information that Biocom Heart Scanner yields. The latter was developed to meet the standards of the European Society of Cardiology and North American Society of Pacing and Electrophysiology. The Freeze-Framer™ uses a treatment procedure radically different from TFT as they attempt to get the person to be rid of negative thoughts by having them think good thoughts and thoughts of love. TFT on the other hand, eliminates the cause of the bad thoughts and it is typically done in minutes, while other procedures may take weeks or months and do not yield the same degree of dramatic results we typically enjoy.

HRV	Percent in High Synch	In the Ideal Zone	Time
Pre-therapy	33%	0%	3:49p.m.
Post-algorithm	54%	0%	3:58p.m.
Post-VT therapy	79%	100%	4:11p.m.

Note that the readings on HRV are reported to be stable over time and it typically takes weeks or months of ordinary work or therapy to change these readings. Here we are working in a *total time frame of mere minutes* (each HRV measure itself was of five minutes duration). There was no attempt to have him think about "nice things."

Another test was given to Jim a month later. His SDNN was 87, his power 3545, and he was within the box. This suggests that the previous treatment has held up.

We now know our successful procedure for treating fibrillation was no fluke or accident. Several TFT trainees have reported, to date, a total of eight cases of fibrillation helped dramatically with TFT Voice Technology™. One of these cases was also in an ICU ward at the time of treatment by telephone.

The simple algorithm improved the heart scores (according to this HRV reading) by 21%. However, the major change brought about by TFT Voice Technology™ is putting the autonomic nervous system into the ideal zone of balance of 100% according to this instrument. *Naturally, all such findings need to be evaluated by a competent cardiologist in terms of guiding the treatment of a particular patient.*

This striking result makes sense as to why the VT treatment was able to help this patient's heart get into the appropriate healthy groove when he was in ICU and suffering additionally from a drug to which he was known to be allergic. It also suggests that an algorithm would not have been sufficient to help dramatically. Later, I obtained a more sophisticated HRV, the Biocom Heart Scanner previously mentioned, which conforms to International Standards of Performance and Jim's score on this instrument will be presented below.

The Precise Treatment

The VT treatment resulted in a far more dramatic result, even though the algorithm improved the situation somewhat. The exact treatment given by VT causal diagnosis was as follows: The letters refer to different acupuncture points, e.g., If = index finger, c = collar bone point, e = under the eye; a = under the arm, etc. 9g indicates to do the nine gamut treatments and sq (for sequence) simply means to repeat the same treatments which came before the nine gamut treatments in each holon.[2] This treatment is *not* an algorithm but was individually determined for this client. It is not likely to help some other person who would probably need to have their own individually diagnosed series of treatments in order to be helped.

If, c, e, a, c, 9g sq
C, tf, eb, sh, c, a, c, 9g sq
E, eb, c, a, c, tf, I, c, a, c, 9g sq

The client tapped each of these points five times. Then he did the nine gamut treatments and then the majors were repeated. Throughout, the client was checked for PR and none occurred during this session.

Ordinarily I am treating psychological problems and measuring the results with an HRV measure. It has increas-

---

[2] A holon simply refers to one series of treatments distinguished by the presence of the nine gamut. In this example, there are three holons. The term "holon" was chosen for it refers to both whole and part. Each treatment is a whole in itself and sometimes is also part of a whole treatment.

ingly become obvious however, as more medical doctors take our training, that TFT can be applied with good results to various medical problems of which this is but one small example.

HRV AND PREVIOUS FINDINGS OF TFT VALIDATED

"HRV studies should enhance our understanding of physiological phenomena, the actions of medications, and disease mechanisms." (Task Force, 1996, p. 1060) A number of findings in TFT are supported by HRV results. For example, we have found a very high relationship between objective improvement in HRV due to TFT treatment and the reported SUD of the client. As the SUD goes down to 1 on the 10-point scale, we see the HRV reflect this change and improvement.

Since TFT is such a powerful and effective treatment and is able to completely eliminate most psychological problems, we are put in the unique position of being able to observe what might make a problem return. We have found that identified toxins allow us to predict with high success what might make an eliminated problem return. The HRV will show a predictable decline when a person ingests or is exposed to a toxin.

We have a phenomenon in TFT we call inertial delay. This is a rare situation when a person is treated with TFT and no further perturbations are showing and yet the client reports no improvement. We usually find after a period of time ranging from minutes to hours (rarely more than one day), the client will report a dramatic improvement. This is unusual in TFT, for most often, change takes place immediately. Occasionally, we have found the same inertial delay with the HRV measurement. Typically, however, just as it is with the SUD, changes on the HRV take place immediately. In general, we can expect inertial delays when toxins and/or advanced age are involved.

HRV IN MEDICAL RESEARCH

EPIDEMIOLOGY

The Framingham Heart Study Group "showed that in a population that was apparently free of coronary heart disease or congestive heart failure, depressed HRV was associated with subsequent cardiac events (angina, myocardial infarction, coronary heart disease death or congestive heart failure." (Yap and Camm, p. 396) (The tests used in these studies were of longer term than we use.) Yap and Camm also report that reduced HRV also predicted an increased risk for all causes of mortality in the elderly population (mean age 72 years).

The role of SDNN (an indicator of the spread of the variability of the heart) was shown to be highly predictive of sudden death. "The results showed patients with low short term RR interval variability (mean during 24 hours of per-minute standard deviation of RR intervals < 25ms (milliseconds) corresponding to SDNN) had a 4.1-fold higher risk for sudden death than patients with higher short-term variability (> 40ms)." (Yap and Camm, p. 397). The authors conclude: "Thus HRV may provide prognostic information beyond that provided by the evaluation of traditional cardiovascular disease risk factors in a seemingly disease free community population." (p. 397) Such predictions of mortality are especially reliable with people who have had a heart attack.

In patients with diabetes mellitus, a reduction in time-domain measures of HRV seems to precede clinical expression of autonomic neuropathy and indicates an adverse prognosis. (Yap and Camm, p. 408) The authors point out that HRV can be important in helping to identify high-risk patients for subsequent management.

Kautzner (1995, pp. 169-170) states HRV is useful in the early diagnosis of diabetes and also for monitoring its progression.

DRUGS AND HRV

"Drugs are a common cause of autonomic dysfunction, often as a side effect" (Mathias and Alam, 1995, p. 22). Tranquilizers also are reported to have a poor effect on HRV.

MORTALITY AND HRV

"In recent years, analysis of heart rate variability (HRV) has become a standard tool for the prediction of cardiac mortality with the general 'rule of thumb' that a reduced variability is a signature for disease and enhanced risk." (Schmidt and Morfill, 1995, p. 87)

Kautzner states that the "reproducibility of HRV indices is far superior to those of other variables that are also known to predict mortality in survivors of myocardial infarction, such as ventricular ectopy or episodes of silent ischemia. Thus, HRV might be preferable for risk stratification studies and for *evaluation of the efficacy of various interventions* [my emphasis]." (p. 170)

Fallen and Kamath (1995) report, regarding sudden cardiac death, that "HRV is a powerful prognosticator of overall mortality." In the chapter on HRV and Sudden Cardiac Death, Singer and Ori, echo the general finding that "low HRV [is] a powerful predictor of all cause mortality." (p. 433) They add:

> Indeed, low HRV, defined in terms of the standard deviation of the mean of all 'normal' RR intervals (i.e., interval between two sequential sinus beats without contained ectopic beats) was found to be a powerful independent predictor of long-term mortality survivors of MI. Similar observations have been reported by others. Indeed, low HRV may be a more powerful predictor of mortality than such standard determinants as left ventricular ejection fraction, wall motion abnormalities, frequency and complexity of ventricular ectopy, standard ECG indices, exercise capacity, and the signal averaged ECG." (p. 434)

They also note, "Combining low HRV (SD measure < 30 milliseconds) and inducibility correctly identified all SCD (sudden cardiac death) survivors who died during a 100-month follow-up." (p. 435) And they add, "Preliminary analysis of data from long term (to 8 years) follow-up of SCD survivors with mortality as the endpoint confirms the strong predictive value of low HRV (SD<30) for recurrence of major arrhythmic events ... five died during the observation period. Of these, four exhibited very low HRV (SD: <20 milliseconds)." (p. 438)

The authors conclude with the strong statement, "Despite these and other caveats, the data support conclusions that HRV determinations represent an independent predictor that greatly facilitates the identification of individuals at increased risk of SCD." (p. 442)

"The absence of variability is a highly significant risk factor for adverse outcomes following acute MI (myocardial infarction), including all cause mortality, arrhythmic, and sudden death." (Bosner and Kleiger, p. 331)

Vanoli et al. (1995) conclude "The lower the HRV, the greater the probability that acute myocardial ischemia results in a dominance of sympathetic reflexes and consequently, in a greater risk for the occurrence of lethal arrhythmias.... A normal HRV after MI reflects a preserved physiological cardiac vagal activity that is protective against ventricular fibrillation." (p. 358)

Casolo (1995) introduces his chapter with the definitive comment: *"It is now generally accepted that heart rate variability (HRV) is reduced in patients with heart failure."* (p. 449)

EXAMPLES OF HRV RESULTS WITH TFT

In measuring HRV we use an instrument called the Heart Scanner. Keep in mind when reviewing our reports that experts in HRV have grown accustomed to seeing only very small, if any, positive changes in HRV scores. Recently, a physician commented, after viewing some of the changes in HRV scores as a result of TFT intervention, that he learned about HRV in medical school but forgot about it since nothing could be done to dramatically improve it. He is very excited to find that in fact HRV can be changed and changed dramatically with TFT. This has renewed his interest in HRV.

I could find in the literature only two reports of improved HRV (SDNN). Both of these involved the use of exercise over time. In one case (Task Force, 1996, p. 1055) reports a study done on dogs given exercise over a six-week period and this improved the SDNN by 74%. A similar study on human males resulted in an improved SDNN score of 69% over an eight-week period (Malfatto, et al pp. 532-538).

One of the scores used to predict mortality is the variation of the periods between beats. "...HRV has become a standard tool for the prediction of cardiac mortality with the general 'rule of thumb' that a reduced variability is a signature for disease and enhanced risk." (Schmidt and Morfill, p. 87) "Numerous studies, carried out using a variety of methodologies, have found low HRV to be a powerful predictor of all cause mortality." (Singer and Ori, p. 433) A measure of this variability is called the SDNN which is the standard deviation (a measure of variability).

Cut-off scores of SDNN below 100, and also below 50 have been used to predict mortality. These scores are used in conjunction with other information, but the SDNN has been found to be the best predictor of mortality not only for heart problems but also for early diagnosis of diabetic neuropathy (Kautzner, p. 170) and for alcoholism. "Several primary neurological disorders including

Parkinson's disease, multiple sclerosis, Guillain-Barre syndrome, and orthostatic hypotension of the Shy-Drage type are associated with altered autonomic function. In some of these disorders, changes in HRV may be an early manifestation of the condition and may be useful in quantifying the rate of disease progression and/or the efficacy of therapeutic interventions." (Task Force, p. 1060)

In our work, we pay attention to three scores on the HRV—the SDNN, the Total Power and the proximity to "the box." Within the box indicates a balanced autonomic nervous system.

MARTIN—BORN WITH A DEFECTIVE HEART

"Martin" is a 44-year-old man who was born with a defective and misplaced heart. He carries a note with him at all times explaining his condition should he be taken into an emergency room. His base scores before treatment were: SDNN=32 (this is below the 50 cut-off point); his pre-treatment power=511. These are very poor scores and reflect his heart problem. Considering the fact of his defective heart, it is astonishing to find how much his scores improve after TFT-VT treatment.

His SDNN of 32 jumps up to 73 (more than double); his power score jumps to a very nice 2170 compared to the extremely low score of 511 prior to TFT-VT treatment. Also, he was not within the box (indicating autonomic nervous system balance) prior to treatment and after treatment his ANS shows balance. He was advised to take a copy of these pre- and post-test results to his cardiologist.

MEDICAL DOCTOR WITH CHRONIC DEPRESSION AND POOR HEALTH

At a recent causal diagnostic training, a 58-year-old physician volunteered to be a demonstration subject. He had suffered from depression for many years and his general health was very poor. Since he did not respond to years of other psychotherapies or depression medications, he simply resigned himself to a life of depression and poor health. He was able to help many others attain good health in his practice but he felt he would never get better. The HRV expert who was present, Peter Julian (a psycho–neuroimmunologist), gave him an HRV prior to treatment. Julian exclaimed that he had never seen such a low power score as **54**! His SDNN was not very good either; it was a dangerously low **32**! I found a psychological reversal present, which had to be corrected or else he would have been impossible to treat. It is possible that if previous therapists knew how to correct this problem, they might have been able to show some results.

Within five minutes I was able to eliminate all traces of depression using standard TFT causal diagnosis. Julian then did another reading and this physician's power score immediately jumped from a record low of **54** to **6596** (in the normal range)—an increase greater than a hundred-fold! His very poor SDNN jumped from a dangerously low **32** to a very desirable **144**! These are the kinds of results that doctors and researchers experienced in HRV find unprecedented.

Psychiatrist with Heart Problem and Worry

In other TFT causal diagnostic trainings, I had the opportunity to treat two more physicians. Each of these doctors had diagnosed heart problems. The first was a 37-year-old psychiatrist who had his own private psychiatric clinic. He requested treatment because he was very worried about the status of his heart, which had been a known problem for five years.

Unfortunately, we did not get a base score before TFT causal diagnostic treatment was done, so it is likely that his HRV scores were worse than indicated here. His SDNN (after TFT causal diagnosis directed therapy) was still a poor **41**. His power after TFT causal diagnosis directed therapy, prior to TFT-VT treatment, was a poor **202** and he was *not within the box*, indicating an imbalance in the ANS.

After VT we got dramatic improvements. His SDNN immediately jumped to **69;** his power score which was a poor **517** (even after treatment!) jumped to **2153**. Prior to the VT treatment he was far from the box (ANS balance) and after the VT he was in the box, showing that his ANS is balanced. Also, his worry, which certainly was not helping the problem but nevertheless is a perfectly normal emotional response, was completely eliminated after the VT treatment. The treatment took about six minutes.

Physician Whose Heart had Stopped

This 36-year-old brilliant physician was victim to a complete heart stoppage three months earlier. Fortunately, he was close to a hospital and they were able to get his heart going again. Prior to TFT-VT his SDNN was a dangerous **16**. This is the lowest SDNN I had ever seen in my few months of doing HRV work. Below 50 is considered risky. His power was also extremely low at **131** and he was far out of the box indicating a severe imbalance in the ANS. After VT treatment we got dramatic improvements. His SDNN, which was a dangerous **16** jumped up to **91**. His power score, which was a serious low of **131** suddenly, expanded to a very nice **3018**. Also, his ANS now shows balance by being within the box.

CONCLUSIONS

The results we report will be very good news to heart patients and their cardiologists. We have shown, thanks to Dr. Royal's discovery regarding HRV and TFT, that we can dramatically improve HRV scores. Prior to this work, only very modest changes were reported due to exercise. Exercise is good in its own right, but TFT and VT can facilitate dramatic improvements in HRV scores in a brief period of time. Recall that exercise improved SDNN by some 70 to 80% in humans and dogs respectively, over many weeks.

These are very small improvements and they took a matter of from six to eight weeks to achieve. The improvements due to TFT are much more powerful and dramatic and increases of 200% are not unusual. Some have improved scores in a ratio of over a hundred times better than before treatment. Also, these changes do not require months of work but are accomplished almost instantly.

Our finding on improving HRV is very promising and like almost of all of TFT the results are unprecedented. It remains to be demonstrated, however, that these very encouraging results get translated into improved quality as well as increased endurance of life. Research and clinical experience strongly suggest this may very well be the case.

CHAPTER 19

NOTES ON MY DISCOVERIES

I am often asked how I made my discoveries. My first answer is that I have been obsessed with learning about psychological problems, especially phobias, ever since I was a child and suffered from many phobias. A fact that greatly intrigued me was that, even as a child, I knew I should not be afraid of these things, but still I could not help it. That my early years were spent in foster homes only increased my desire to know more about such problems. In more recent professional years, as phobias became rather simple for me to cure, I began to explore other psychological problems, starting with trauma response and today covering the whole gamut of psychological problems. We are now beginning to enter the domain of healing for all kinds of problems, especially medical problems for people who do not respond to conventional approaches, or who respond too slowly for practical purposes.

We often hear that discovery is an accident but this misses the essential aspect of true discovery, for accidents happen all the time to everyone, but significant discovery is rare. As Winston Churchill said, "People stumble over the truth frequently, but most just pick themselves up and carry on as if nothing happened."

I once asked a successful composer how he came up with his compositions. He felt very sheepish answering but he knew that my question was serious. He said, "Roger, this will really sound ridiculous to you but the best answer I can give you is that it is just like going to the bathroom [a polite version of his exact words]."

I believe Arthur M. Young, who invented the Bell helicopter and was a brilliant thinker, explains best why it is so difficult for originators to give a simple answer to discovery or creativity. Young (1976, 1979b, 1980) holds that discovery is a form of first cause, and first cause by definition defies all explanation. Fleming discovered penicillin by "accident," it is often claimed, but the question is how to explain the many other lab workers who for years had the same kind of accidents and felt their petri dish samples were ruined but did not discover penicillin.

A similar example is the discovery of vulcanized rubber. Goodyear was looking for a solution to a problem and thus, Young (1940, p. 176) says, it was *purpose* that was responsible for this discovery and purpose is another ineffable first cause.[1] Young also talks about the importance of recognition or recognizing a solution when it is

---

[1] Young says that "necessity may be the mother of invention, but purpose is the father."

there. Recognition that an answer is correct is a vital aspect of discovery. Young points out that "pots boiling over do not imply rubber tires, or even rubber." The cause was Goodyear, whose intention to find a way of improving raw rubber had led him to cooking it on the stove. It is true that there were other causes (hot stove, accident, etc.) but the first cause—Goodyear's intention—is the only one that implies improved rubber and was responsible for his *recognition* of the solution when it accidentally occurred. Young goes on to explain that first cause need not be without temporal antecedents. "What makes it first cause is that the antecedents do not imply the result."

DISCOVERIES AT THE CONFLUENCE

"It is almost a tradition in the history of science that the discoveries that open up the finest perspectives lie at the confluence of several disciplines." (Jacques, p. 30) For example, Darwin and Wallace, the co-discoverers of natural selection (the theory of evolution), both read and were greatly influenced by the economic and mathematical work of Thomas Malthus. (Milner, 1990)

The therapy I call Thought Field Therapy (TFT) lies at the confluence of the quite diverse fields of clinical psychology, applied kinesiology (chiropractic), acupuncture, quantum physics[2] and biology. I was not trained in acupuncture, but merely explored what I read about it. I often say that if I had been trained I probably would not have made the discoveries I was able to make, for I went

---

[2] The fundamental concept in my work, the perturbation, bridges the fields of psychology, biology and quantum physics.

on this adventure alone. This might be called the "power of ignorance."

My work is sometimes characterized by others as a combination of acupuncture and Applied Kinesiology. Though partially accurate, this is quite misleading. Acupuncture has been around for five or six thousand years and, as far as I can determine, offers nothing close to the kind of treatment power I have been able to squeeze out of my version of this discipline—Callahan Techniques® Thought Field Therapy or CTTFT—has ever before been accomplished. This new power is due to a combination of my separate discoveries:

1. The gradual development of my *causal diagnosis* procedure.

2. The discovery of psychological reversal (my first discovery in TFT) and its correction—the success rate of any therapy is necessarily limited without the PR correction knowledge. I estimate that the success rate is limited by approximately 40% without the PR correction.

3. The thought field itself. From the beginning I had the client *"think about the problem"* which caused the appropriate thought field to be attuned and thereby allowed specific tailor-made treatment addressed to a particular problem possible. Psychological reversals, for example, are specific to certain thought fields, as are the perturbations that need to be treated.

When you go to your acupuncturist, your applied kinesiologist, your physician, your dentist, your massage therapist—it makes no difference to them what you think about when they treat you—unless they have been influenced by my procedures. This fact makes our work far more complex (as well as precise and specific) than any of the above disciplines since we can have an almost infinite number of thought fields to be attuned and treated.

A number of acupuncturists who also do psychotherapy have taken my training. One of them said to me, "Why didn't I think of this?" A psychologist, who is also a trained acupuncturist reported that he had treated approximately twenty-five severely depressed patients with acupuncture and stated that almost all of them had shown at least some degree of improvement. He added, however, that the recovery did not endure unless the acupuncture was accompanied by "appropriate psychotherapeutic care."

I work, for example, with severely depressed clients who have not responded either to conventional psychotherapy and/or medications and I typically and dramatically help them within minutes. If the depression that I eliminated should return, I would not consider referring them for conventional psychotherapy or medications. I would immediately run tests with my causal diagnosis procedures which would inform me of the specific reason for the return of the problem.

If I were unable to help the client, then and only then would I consider referring them for some other therapy or for medication. However, it is an extremely rare event when my treatment cannot help a client.

I sometimes hear that acupuncture is helpful in treating addictions but I claim—and my trainees and I can easily demonstrate—that it is possible with CTTFT not only to help addictions, but to do something that almost all workers in the field of addiction believe is impossible—to eliminate all traces of acute withdrawal, even in heroin addicts. We do this regularly with alcoholics, crack addicts, smokers, and even food addicts.[3]

Causal Diagnosis with EAV

One professional who is skilled in acupuncture and has an EAV (Electroacupuncture by Voll) machine reported that he typically had trouble eliminating migraine headaches. After learning my causal diagnostic procedures, he did something very interesting and original. Instead of using the standard EAV procedure, he used it to find the sequence of points relevant to the problem after having the patient think of the problem. He then eliminated the migraine using the EAV!

Applied Kinesiology

Psychologists, psychiatrists, and other psychotherapists have explored Applied Kinesiology (AK) for working with psychological problems. To the best of my knowl-

---

[3] When I first developed my addiction algorithm, for example, I treated 100 call-in guests who were craving various substances successfully before I had my first failure. Later, the success rate for the addiction algorithm leveled out at about 80 to 90%.

edge, even though AK had been around for over two decades prior to the development of my work, none of these professionals has developed anything close to the power of the procedures I developed.

Part of the problem of some pioneers who combined psychology and AK was that they relied only on the outcome of the muscle test for evidence—this was their bottom line. This is a huge error, for it allows one to wrongly support already existing erroneous ideas, notions and theories.

My work differed in that I did not allow any pre-existing theories to have an influence on my entirely new work. *I considered all results of AK testing to be provisional until confirmed by tangible external evidence.* For example, when a client reported a problem reduced significantly or was completely gone *then, and only then, did I know that I was on the right track* and that my diagnoses and subsequent treatments were on line with reality. The people I saw use muscle testing for psychological problems years ago were completely satisfied with whatever results the test showed. The muscle test can be extremely unreliable and operators, alas, even subconsciously, can make results accord with their beliefs or expectations. Hence bias prevents actual discovery. I have seen many instances of this fatal shortcoming.

After I developed my procedures, a number of other professionals incorporated some of my discoveries in order to develop something similar, but still not as demonstrably powerful as the comprehensive procedures I developed.[4] Now I am fully aware that this may not a politically correct kind of statement but it is accurate. Since these facts are generally unknown, it is necessary for me to make them clear.

It is just as unethical to minimize a finding as it is to exaggerate a finding. It is crucial in science to strive for accuracy, neither minimizing nor exaggerating findings. I have found that some of my trainees, expecting few to believe how powerful these treatments actually are, tend to minimize the extreme power of these treatments.

PASTEUR ON DISCOVERY

I have always been fond of the famous quote by Pasteur that identifies an essential feature of discovery: *"In the field of observation, chance favors the prepared mind."* (Jacques, p. 125) Pasteur said this in an official address delivered at the Lille Faculty of Science on December 7, 1854. Jacques suggests adding another statement from the same source: "Knowing what to wonder at is the first movement of the mind toward discovery." The latter quote is more profound than the former since it is antecedent to the former in the discovery process.

I am fond of quoting and personally resonate to Einstein's response to the question when he was asked how he made his spectacular discoveries about nature: "By thinking of practically nothing else." Although correct, this charming quote does not tell us what goes on in

---

[4] We regularly in CTTFT help clients that no one else can help. When some other procedure can help clients that we cannot help, then we will know that there is something worth knowing.

the process of discovery. A more detailed and eloquent general hint of what is involved in grasping what I consider my major discovery—the discovery of the control system for all healing (not just psychological problems—is given in D. Blatner's (1997) marvelous book about Pi:[5]

> Suppose I give you two sequences of numbers, such as...
>
> 78539816339774830961566084...and 1, -1/3, +1/5, -1/7, +1/9, -1/11, +1/13, -1/15
>
> ...If I asked you, Simplico, what the next number of the first sequence is, what would you say?
>
> I could not tell you. I think it is a random sequence and that there is no law in it.
>
> And for the second sequence?
>
> That would be easy. It must be +1/17.
>
> Right. But what would you say if I told you that the first sequence is also constructed by a law and this law is in fact identical with the one you have just discovered in the second sequence?
>
> This does not seem probable to me.
>
> But it is indeed so, since the first sequence is simply the beginning of the decimal fraction [expansion] of the sum of the second. Its value is pi/4.

---

[5]   The quotation is originally by J.M.Jauch (*Are Quanta Real?*) as quoted in Douglas Hofstadter's *Godel. Escher, Bach.*

You are full of such mathematical tricks, but I do not see what this has to do with abstraction and reality.

The relationship with abstraction is easy to see. The first sequence looks random unless one has developed through a process of abstraction a kind of filter which sees a simple structure behind the apparent randomness [my emphasis].

It is exactly in this manner that laws of nature are discovered. Nature presents us with a host of phenomena which appear mostly as chaotic randomness until we select some significant events, and abstract from their particular, irrelevant circumstances so they become idealized. Only then can they exhibit their true structure in full splendor.

The filter referred to here would be what I call causal diagnosis. This filter led to discovery of the continued revelations of the coding for the healing system which are alluded to in the quotations below.

It's God's job to hide things and man's job to find them.

Sir Francis Bacon
Founder of Western Science

What scientists do is little different from what Talmudists do: There is a coded message, [you] find the code.

Albert Libchaber
Scientific American

The benevolence of Natural Law lies in assuring us that...miracles are open to us, but it does not extend to telling us how to accomplish them; it is for us to discover the keys, the encodings and decodings, by which they can be brought to pass.

Robert Rosen
Theoretical Biologist

Lastly, and most importantly, all my discoveries were continually checked by clinical experiments. The fact that Nature has provided for almost immediate results in this domain of work made the process much easier than if healing should always require the passage of much time. If the latter were the case, I might have had to wait weeks, months or years before knowing the result of any of my novel efforts. Immediate feedback[6] of the results was a major factor that contributed greatly to the rapid accumulation of my various discoveries.

I once compared this process to someone throwing darts at a dartboard but receiving no feedback on how close the dart comes to the target. This is the actual state in conventional psychotherapy. Obviously, one can do better if one can get immediate feedback on the success or failure of any procedure. Think of this advantage alone— *we do not have to experiment with worthless procedures for years before knowing they are worthless.*

---

[6] It is rare that a change is not immediate, but once in a few hundred cases we find that someone may take an hour or more before the treatment takes effect. I call this inertial delay, for I believe that the delay is caused by the literal mass involved in people who are sensitive to some common foods, drinks or other items.

Are there more discoveries to be made in CTTFT? Yes is a safe answer. Just within the last year I made two new discoveries which have significantly increased the power of Voice Technology™ (VT), which already was quite close to perfect! One of these discoveries allowed me to treat a few people successfully who would have been untreatable prior to these discoveries and the other provided for more convenience and speed in the treatment of difficult cases. These discoveries have been tested and found powerful by other VT-trained professionals.

There are major discoveries to be made on how to increase the power of treatment for people whose systems are toxic (either by ingested toxins, toxic exposures, or infections). We already know a lot about this domain and enjoy considerable success, but there is room for improvement. As one can see in the chapter on Causal Diagnosis, our results in VT are pushing an upper limit, very close to perfection, but still short of perfection.[7] This gap presents a continuing challenge to the creative people who are trained in and work at the VT level.

It takes more than a mere claim to establish a valid discovery. Claims are cheap and are commonly made by some pretentious individuals. I sometimes hear about so-called improvements in my procedures and look forward to their being established, but have yet to have any valid demonstration supporting them. In CTTFT a claim is impressive if it allows us to help someone we could not help

---

[7] Rational perfection, in this context, does not require 100% success but only closer to that ideal than is currently possible. Any procedure that can improve our results in speed and/or effectiveness takes us closer to our goal of having as high a success rate as is possible.

before, or if we can help someone with more speed and/ or effectiveness than was possible before. I am certain that with time there will be others who will make some original, substantive contributions. We now have a few people trained at our top level whose work is promising, and we look forward to the results of their continuing efforts.

What is required in establishing a new discovery in this domain is to show that the discovery allows an already very high success rate to be raised. This is not so easy, it is not impossible. The contribution must show that it can do work which the already existing body of knowledge and procedures I have developed cannot do; or it will be helpful if it can be shown that the work can be done easier and more effectively. It was far easier to make new discoveries in the very early days of the development of this work since the success rate at that time was far lower (3%) than it is today (98 to 99%).[8] Now, with such high power and success readily available, it is not at all easy to make significant new discoveries, though we are always on the lookout for authentic new discoveries and will be very excited when it happens.

One of our great scientists, Nobel Laureate Richard Feynman (1967), put the issue squarely and clearly (as he so often did): "We have to find a new view of the world that has to agree with everything that is known, but disagree in its predictions somewhere, otherwise it is not interesting. And in that disagreement *it must agree with*

---

[8] The two latest discoveries plus some important findings re nutritional support are pushing the success beyond 99%.

nature. [If one] can do this, you have made a great discovery. It is very nearly impossible, but not quite...."

Observe how the principle of "agreeing with nature" is demonstrated in the dramatic example below. This example, is just one among very many similar ones in our files. Following is a helpful analogy by Dr. Stephen Daniel, FPPR, VT.

Specificity and TFT

Dr. Roger Callahan made many remarkable discoveries in the development of TFT. Perhaps the most impressive is the specificity of TFT. Let me explain: Last week I was at an exhibit for holistic practitioners in my area. I sat at a table with two trained acupuncturists. They each had an issue that they had been unable to heal with needles. I offered to treat them on the spot and rapidly cleared both of them of their long-standing problems that were unresponsive to their efforts.

They asked me why I thought TFT worked when acupuncture didn't. "Aren't we both working on the same meridians?"

Here was my response: "The oldest, wisest acupuncturist is like the oldest, wisest locksmith. The locksmith, when confronted with a new and unknown safe, brings his years of wisdom and his understanding of codes to the task. Because he knows a lot about the makes and models of safes, and knows the most common combinations, he will eventually figure out how to open a safe. There will still be a few safes he cannot open.

Now imagine that I come along and can talk to the safe, and the safe gives me the exact numbers in the exact sequence. This is what happens in TFT. In acupuncture the therapist is using tried-and-true formulas, but they are still formulas. I, on the other hand, using the *specificity* of TFT, through causal diagnosis, can talk to the body, and the body reveals to me exactly where to tap and in what specific sequence. Specificity revealed by causal diagnosis, as well as the concept of reversal are two of the major reasons why TFT is so incredibly far ahead of any other form of healing.

OTHER DISCOVERIES

Psychological Reversal (PR)—My first discovery, PR, is perhaps the single most powerful treatment. Done alone, it can and has accomplished many positive changes. Any treatment which uses pr correction will automatically obtain a higher success rate.

A few years after PR, I discovered Mini-PR, which allows for more complete treatment. Also, I have discovered some other variants of PR which help contribute to our astonishing success rate. Any treatment which incorporates PR knowledge will have a higher success rate than otherwise.

Collarbone Breathing—The old AK treatment for switching was called cross-crawl. Dr. Walther was never satisfied with this dubious treatment and somehow came up with a cranial treatment which corrected the problem without cross-crawl and the treatment is called the Cross K-

27[9] Treatment. In order to do cranial manipulation, which can be dangerous if not done correctly, highly specialized knowledge is required. The evidence suggests that my collarbone breathing treatment accomplishes the same result. My discovery was that tapping the gamut point while going through this complex (compared to our other treatments) procedure would do the job so that a lay person could carry out this important treatment.

Discovery of Sequence of P's—In my first days of TFT, two decades ago, I was fortunate to find that only one (but it had to be the proper one) point (or perturbation) was needed to cure a phobia (under the eye) and trauma (the beginning of the eyebrow). However, I quickly found that the success rate of this procedure was quite low. For this reason I searched and found that in some cases a series of points were required in the correct order and that this would help more people. Today, through Voice Technology™ (VT), where we specialize in helping people that no one else is able to help, we sometimes find a very large series of points that need addressing. Sometimes we find many hundreds of points required. We know the order is crucial because we in VT work successfully with people who have tried random tapping of all the points many times with no good result. It is not until we determine the correct sequence that we get our powerful results in such cases.

---

9   In acupuncture, the 27th point on the kidney meridian is located just under the collar bone. What I call the "collarbone point" is the K27.

The Nine Gamut Series—Eye movements were used in diagnosis in Neuro-Linguistic Training (NLP), for some diagnostic purposes in AK and in Feldenkreis method. What I did was to confirm that the position of the eyes would indeed diagnostically reveal a problem in the system, but my discovery was that the ubiquitous gamut spot, when tapped, would provide a correction for the problem which yielded immediate and obvious reductions in the problem.

Causal Diagnosis—To my knowledge, I am the first who publicly claimed a cure for psychological problems (Callahan, 1985). Through recognizing the cure, I was gradually able to see that I had also developed what for the first time in psychiatry and psychology could reasonably be called a causal diagnosis. What has been called diagnosis is actually descriptive or nosological procedures of placing people into categories. That is not what my procedure is at all. CTTFT causal diagnosis reveals the specific causes of any particular problem. It is this procedure which is responsible for my high success rate.

Architecture of the Procedures—Often overlooked is the fact that I discovered a certain structure to the treatments which helps contribute to the high success we enjoy. That structure consists of doing what I call the majors (eyebrow, eye, collar bone), followed by the nine gamut, and then the majors are repeated. A briefer way to express this is: major—nine gamut—major. Obviously not everyone needs the whole architecture for tapping—one point for a small number of people was effective. For most people we strongly recommend the structure, which is common and will contribute to a higher success rate.

HEART RATE VARIABILITY (HRV)

I believe that no therapy in the future will be considered valid unless it passes the HRV test. Dr. Fuller Royal introduced me to this important physiological measure of, among other things, a clear indicator of the status of the autonomic nervous system. We have had four independent HRV operators located in different areas—Nevada, Colorado, Norway and Japan. All have proclaimed that they have never seen any treatment with the power to balance the autonomic nervous system, as measure by HRV, as does CTTFT. The HRV operator in Norway, who had done 10,000 HRV's:

> John Hetelid, an expert in the field of Heart Rate Variability testing was the next to speak. He expressed his own astonishment at the instantaneous impact of CTTFT on HRV—apparently on testing TFT for the first time he was convinced that there was an error in the data he obtained. Only when the test was repeated with the same result did he believe what he had witnessed! Much data was then presented that confirmed CTTFT's capability. (Graham, Ian, 1999)

APPENDIX A

TFT GLOSSARY

ADDICTION An addict does what most modern psychiatrists recommend: "When anxious, take a tranquilizer." The typical addict chooses from a far wider variety of tranquilizers than the psychiatrist who is limited to FDA-approved medications. No such restriction burdens the average serious addict. A behavioral addiction serves a similar purpose to the anxious person as a substance, i.e., it masks anxiety. Behavioral addictions consist of such things as body picking, hair pulling, nail biting, hand washing, and the disorder known as Obsessive Compulsive Disorder (OCD).

ADDICTIVE URGE The immediate desire, urge or compulsion to engage in or consume an addictive substance or engage in an addictive behavior. It is powered by a growing intensity in anxiety and the consequent need for a tranquilizer. It is the TFT position that all tranquilizers merely mask anxiety; they do not eliminate the cause. An effective masking tranquilizer becomes addictive; therefore any effective mask of anxiety is potentially addictive. TFT-addictive urge treatment typically eliminates every trace of' addictive urge, even for heroin, pain pills, alcohol, nicotine, and crack. TFT treatment addresses the underlying cause of addiction and does not merely mask addictive urge. As Thomas Szasz puts it, "Giving methadone to a heroin addict is like giving scotch to a bourbon addict."

ADDICTIVE-URGE TREATMENT The thought field therapy procedure for reducing intense anxiety and thereby reducing or eliminating the addictive urge and the withdrawal symptoms associated with addiction.

ALGORITHM R.M. Youngson (1994) defines an algorithm as "a sequence of instructions to be followed with the intention of finding a solution to a problem. Each step must specify precisely what action is to be taken, and although there may be many alternate routes through the algorithm, there is only one start point and one end point." (p. 232) The start point in TFT is usually a SUD of 10 and the end point is a 1. In TFT an algorithm is a recipe or formula for treatment of a particular problem discovered by TFT diagnosis that has been tested on many people and has been found to have a high success rate. An algorithm permits an untrained person to readily enter the domain of TFT treatment success.

AMYGDALA An almond-shaped portion of the brain that is receiving much attention by some of the most accomplished researchers in psychology. They believe that this portion of the brain will ultimately be shown to be the basis for controlling anxiety and other problems (LeDoux, 1995). There is no current support for this promise of ultimate control and there is not likely to be any since, like the chemical theory, we believe the researchers are looking in the wrong direction. The meridian system can be readily shown to be the fundamental control system for the negative emotions when it is used according to the encodings and other discoveries of TFT.

ANTICIPATORY ANXIETY A myth. Anticipatory anxiety is identical to tuning into a perturbed thought field. It may be called anticipatory when the tuning takes place prior to engaging in a feared situation.

ANXIETY A type of vague, intense fear which is pervasive, nonfocused, and extremely unpleasant.

APEX PROBLEM The apex problem is when a successfully treated client accurately reports that the problem is gone but is unable to see that the therapy did the job. It is a robust tendency—it could be called a compulsion—for treated clients or even scientific observers of therapy, to give "explanations" of the treatments which careful thought reveal to be totally inappropriate and irrelevant. These include distraction, hypnosis, and placebo. Even therapists who observe TFT will suggest this, though there is no basis in research for such a claim. Typically, professional observers of the demonstrated results of TFT will not *ask* but rather will compulsively *tell* the therapist their (usually totally irrelevant) version of what took place. Many TFT-trained therapists insist on recording a therapy session because some clients "forget" that they had a problem after the rapid successful therapy. We call this phenomenon the apex problem because the mind is *not* operating at the apex or top level. When confronted with something as strange and revolutionary as TFT, the mind has trouble grasping and understanding these new treatments. Most of us attempt to avoid such work and mistakenly attempt to fit our observation into something we *believe* we understand. The identification of the apex problem has scientific utility in that it refines prediction, i.e., we predict that the client will report improvement and further predict that he is not likely to credit the therapy for the improvement.

ATAVISM A term in biology that refers to a throwback to an earlier ancestral form (e.g., a human baby born with a tail or extra nipples). In TFT the term refers to the return of a psychological problem, within the individual's lifetime, which has been eliminated by therapy or has been subsumed naturally due to maturity (see Neoteny). Biological atavisms have been shown to occur under toxic influence, radiation, etc. In a similar fashion, we find that toxins can generate the return of a problem that has either been successfully treated or eliminated through maturation. An example of the latter is a person who, through normal development, outgrew the fear of heights, which is universal in crawling infants, but the fear suddenly returned at some later time in life. A fear of heights that suddenly returns in adulthood, or a problem that had been removed through successful treatment, then returns, would be considered atavistic. These are rare events, but in TFT we have identified exogenous causes of atavisms and can carry out preventive steps.

CAUSALITY A basic concept in physics and chemistry and not much used in psychology. TFT requires the introduction of causality for we have overwhelming evidence that our causal diagnostic procedures reveal the fundamental causes of disturbing emotions.

CHEMICAL THEORY The theory that holds that chemical changes in the brain and nervous system are the *basic* causes of disturbed emotions. Although there are certainly chemical and hormonal facts concurrent with negative emotions, we propose that the chemistry is secondary or tertiary to the more fundamental perturbations (see below).

COMPULSION A powerful urge or desire which is extremely difficult or impossible to resist.

CONCATENATION A connection in a link or chain. Codes for subsumption of perturbations are concatenated by diagnosis. DNA was uninteresting until Watson and Crick found that sequences were important. This meant a code or software.

CONTROL SYSTEM A small system that governs or controls a larger system. The control system on an automobile, for example, consists of the accelerator, the steering wheel, the gears, and the brake. The control system for the negative emotions resides in the body's little-known but demonstrably real energy or meridian system.

CURE The eradication or significant reduction of a problem. The correction or relief of a disturbing condition. A complete cure means that no symptoms or aspects of the problem remain after treatment. After a cure we track for endurance. If there is no toxic exposure, or other extreme stress, the cure will likely endure over time.

DIAGNOSIS The art of discovering the fundamental causal constituents responsible for a psychological problem. Conventional psychological diagnosis is typically directed toward classifying a person according to symptoms, with little or no direct implication for treatment. Diagnosis in TFT is directed toward identifying the specific causal entities of the problem for the purpose of treatment (see Perturbations below). TFT diagnosis does not consist of bestowing mere empty descriptive terms, but rather is a *dynamic revelation of causal constituents*. Diagnosis may be considered to be a translation of the encoded language of the Negative Emotions into a form that can be addressed in treatment. (See Language of negative emotions below). There is a demonstrable isomorphic relationship between the perturbations as diagnosed and those in the perturbed thought field.

ENERGY SYSTEM A palpable, tangible series of electric or electromagnetic circuitry or meridians throughout the whole body, which appear to act as a governing force in healing and growth. These electric systems have been scientifically established at various research centers. The energy, or meridian system, acts as a control system for the negative emotions. The reality of these systems is made quite apparent with TFT.

FEAR A highly focused, unpleasant emotion that provokes avoidance. It is a natural capacity of higher chordates that helps protect the individual by motivating the avoidance of danger (see Anxiety and Phobia).

FIELD A dictionary definition of field is "a complex of forces that serve as causative agents in human behavior." More generally, a field is an invisible non-material structure in space that has an effect upon matter. Michael Faraday, a self-educated genius, introduced *field* to science. Einstein gives credit to Faraday in his Nobel acceptance speech and stated that if Faraday had gone to college he probably never would have been able to invent the revolutionary concept of the field, which is fundamental to Einstein's and Maxwell's work in physics. For example, the gravity field is seen to cause the ocean to curve around the gravity-curved earth. In the psychological realm, the thought field is considered to be more like an electromagnetic pattern on video or recording tape, i.e., it is neither chemical nor cognitive in its basic constituency. Today, many scientists consider that everything is composed of fields. "The visible world is neither matter nor spirit but the invisible organization of energy," wrote physicist Heinz Pagels. The term *morphic field* was introduced into biology to explain the shape and form of living things by Alexander Gurwitsch (Russia) in 1922, and independently in 1925 by Paul Weiss (Vienna). Waddington in England, in the 1950s, added the concept of the *chreode* (necessary path) to the biological field that incorporated time in embryological development. Rupert Sheldrake introduced the concept of morphic resonance between similar fields that can account for how instinctual information is transmitted. Such information cannot be contained in the DNA and can only be learned in interaction with the environment. In 1991, the concept of perturbation (see below) was introduced to account for the fundamental causal aspect of negative emotions. If a bee is placed in a strong magnetic field, his hivemates will no longer recognize him.

GAMUT SPOT A commonly used treatment spot in TFT which is located on the back of either hand.

GAMUT TREATMENTS A series of nine treatments which are done while tapping the gamut spot on the back of the hand. This series of treatments, which is useful to see as a unit, is used for treating most problems. Six of the nine treatments involve certain eye movements and eye positions. The other three, we believe, activate right (humming) and left (counting) brain. We have learned that it is important to do the humming, followed by the counting, and then repeat the humming.

HABIT A behavior routine carried out without conscious awareness; similar to instinct. Habit allows us to focus our attention on other issues. Habits can be confused with addictions, but are distinguished from addiction by being *relatively* easy to change if conscious attention is focused on the issue. Addictions are difficult and habits are easy, but the latter requires continuing conscious attention in order to be modified. Addictions require effective therapy and then may become rather easy to eliminate.

HOLON Holon refers to an architectural feature of TFT that refers to the therapy sequence: majors—nine gamut—majors. Most problems require but one holon but some complex problems may require 40 or more holons before relief is experienced. Each therapy sequence of majors—nine gamut—majors, is defined as a holon.

INERTIAL DELAY This term refers to an unusual situation in TFT where the client shows no perturbations in diagnosis and yet the problem or some degree of the problem appears to remain. After the passage of time, varying from minutes to hours, the client then reports the problem gone. Since we expect a problem to be gone almost instantly in TFT, we take special notice of delays.

INERTIAL LADEN Psychological problems may be characterized as being less inertial laden than physical problems. We refer to the obvious fact that physically inherited characteristics, such as eye color, are more physical and therefore inertial laden (with mass) than psychological characteristics, such as memory or information. An audiotape itself may be said to be inertial laden, while the information contained in the magnetic field imprinted upon it is much less laden with inertia. This low inertial feature intrinsic to psychological problems is the major reason that complete cure is commonplace in our psychotherapy and also becomes so astonishingly simple and rapid once the encodings of nature are understood.

ISOMORPHISM Isomorphism is defined in dictionaries as a math term: a one-to-one relation onto the map between two sets which preserves the relations existing between elements in its domain; something identical with or similar to something else in form or structure. This term in TFT summarizes and expresses the basic finding that there is a strong one-to-one relationship between perturbations (diagnosed) in the thought field and specific energy median points on the body.

LANGUAGE OF NEGATIVE EMOTIONS The causal aspect of the negative emotions exists in encoded form. Language refers to the particular perturbations (P's) in their specific, discrete order, which generate negative emotions. The requirement for specific order is similar to a combination lock; if the wrong order is offered it doesn't work. P's are often contained in certain common orders for specific problems, which makes it possible to determine algorithms or common recipes for many psychological problems. Each negative emotion exists in encoded form which accurate TFT causal diagnosis reveals. The other encoded language appearing in nature is that of DNA, which determines the structure of proteins.

LEVELS OF TFT PROFICIENCY *Level one* is the algorithm, which is quite simple and can be learned by video and/or seminar and can be done by anyone who studies the material carefully. *Level two* is the approved algorithm training seminar by a certified TFT instructor who has completed diagnostic training. We also recommend that anyone who works with people study the relevant algorithm video. *Level three* is what we call the diagnostic level, where the individual is trained in the more complex TFT diagnostic procedures and becomes certified after completion of diagnostic training. This level trains the practitioner to diagnose and treat with greater success, and to address a greater number of problems in the office than the first or algorithmic level. Training at the diagnostic level is done in three steps. Step A is a combination of video, and audiotape instruction, writings; Step B is a seminar where the trainee gets hands-on, in-person instruction; and Step C includes six months of supervision by telephone with the Voice Technology™ (see below). The certified diagnostic level person also gains a much higher degree of understanding of theory and is empowered to causally diagnose and treat most psychological problems with a high degree of success. As in all the professions, continual practice is necessary to keep skills current. *Level four* is the Voice Technology™, which requires training and equipment beyond the diagnostic level, but requires the diagnostic level of training before becoming eligible. This level is a significant advance above the previous two levels. The Voice Technology™ training goes on for three years as needed. It is open only to those certified at the diagnostic level. The Voice Technology™ has the highest precision and success rate and allows one to treat effectively by telephone, which opens up worldwide potential markets for practice and consultations. As in all professions those who *practice* the treatments gain the highest degree of competence.

MAGNETITE Joseph L. Kirschvink, Professor of Geobiology at Caltech, discovered the presence of magnetite throughout the human brain. On November 5, 1992, Joanne and I saw him demonstrate this startling fact in a lecture; a magnet placed near brain samples under the microscope clearly showed the particles of magnetite. Keeping in mind that nature is rarely frivolous, one wonders: What is magnetite doing in the human brain? Could it be there to be responsive to emg fields?

MAJORS A term, which refers to the treatments that use certain meridian points, such as under the eye, under the arm, beginning of eyebrow, etc. The term "majors" distinguishes this aspect of the treatment procedure from the nine gamut, floor-to-ceiling eye roll, the collarbone breathing, and the psychological reversal treatments. The major treatments occur before and are typically repeated after the nine gamut procedure.

NEOTENY A problem or condition due to the lack of full development. For example, all infants (and all land-based chordates) are born with an instinctive fear of heights, which ripens when the neonate begins to crawl or move under its own initiative. Acrophobia is usually outgrown with normal development. A person who has been afraid of heights since childhood is considered in TFT theory to be "neotenous."

PERTURBATION (P) A perturbation is a proposed entity in the thought field. The P is viewed as the fundamental and basic cause of all negative emotions. A perturbation is the unit of fundamental causation of a negative emotion and, in a wonderful blessing of nature, correlates with specific energy points (called alarm points) on the body. Successful therapy subsumes or reduces the impact of P's in the thought field (see below). A P is a subtle, but clearly isolable aspect of a thought field that is responsible for triggering all negative emotions. No P, no negative emotion. The P is the generating structure that determines the chemical, hormonal, nervous system, cognitive, and brain activity commonly associated with negative emotions. It is an intrinsic and necessary part (but *not* the fundamental cause) of the negative emotions. The perturbation contains the *active information,* which triggers negative emotions. Bohm and Hiley (1993) describe their pivotal concept in quantum physics: "[W]e have introduced a concept that is new in the context of physics—a concept that we shall call active information. The basic idea of active information is that a form having very little energy enters into and directs a much greater energy. The activity of the latter is in this way given a form similar to that of the smaller energy." (p. 35) The process described here for quantum theory appears to fit the notions of numerous investigators into the bioenergy realm as the process by which biological control systems operate. One may understand the relevance of the TFT usage of "active information" in that the microstate of the perturbations generate the macrostate that the person feels when depressed, angry, anxious, etc. Successful psychotherapy is the transformation (or subsumption) of this active informational microstate (perturbation) that results in the commonly observed and successfully predicted elimination of the negative emotions in TFT.

PHOBIA A persistent fear of a harmless object or situation. Most people with phobias are very much aware of the irrationality of the fear, which only adds to their difficulty. The knowledge that the fear makes no sense does not reduce the fear, but merely adds embarrassment to the bad feeling. The commonly held idea that the problem is due to a lack of courage is without any foundation whatsoever and shows a fundamental lack of understanding of this kind of psychological problems.

PUBLIC DEMONSTRATIONS In the early days of psychotherapy, treatments were secretive. Even today one may hear strong claims for success, but it is rare that public demonstrations are given. (A gentleman in his late 80s went for a physical examination because he was losing interest in sex. His doctor pronounced him in good health and told him that his decline was a normal function of aging. The man said, "But doctor, my friend Sam is 90 years old and he says that he has sex every night!" The doctor replied, *"You can say that too!"*) In secrecy it is safe to make strong claims. We have done public demonstrations since TFT was first discovered. Most people, much to my surprise, do not appear to grasp the scientific significance of a public demonstration. *The Wall Street Journal* of Monday, January 29, 1996, page A9A mentions public demonstrations in an article on the controversial subject of cold fusion. In "A Bottle Rekindles Scientific Debate About the Possibility of Cold Fusion," Jerry E. Bishop wrote: "The Patterson cell might have been dismissed as easily as other reputed 'cold fusion apparatus.' But Mr. Reding and his colleagues have been bold enough to demonstrate it at three technical conferences in the last nine months. Most cold-fusionists are reluctant to show off their devices, because they are never sure whether or when they will work." In TFT we never know whether our public demonstrations will work, but we do know that the odds are on our side.

PSYCHOLOGICAL REVERSAL (PR) A state or condition that blocks natural healing and prevents otherwise effective treatments from working. Evidence for the state of PR is revealed when an otherwise effective treatment does nothing—then after the PR is corrected, the same treatment suddenly works. A person may be fine in most domains of his life and be PR in just one or a selected few. The PR state is usually accompanied by negative attitudes and self-sabotaging behavior. A most interesting symptom of PR is that expressed concepts are often reversed 180 degrees (e.g., a person will say "south" when he means "north," but will not say "east" or "west"). It seems to relate to a fundamental aspect of direction (chirality, polarized light, etc.) in elemental reality. A similar and related symptom of PR is getting numbers or letters out of order. The upside-down and backward writing of dyslexia is due to the PR. In most of us, PR is a temporary condition. A research study (Blaich, 1988) compared a number of rather complicated and specialized treatments designed to improve human performance; the rapid (10 seconds) and simple treatment for PR was by far the most effective in improving performance in reading speed and comprehension. We find the presence of PR on treatment effect to be quite lawful and predictable. The concept of PR is relevant to all applied fields, a vital phenomenon to successful treatment. The treatments would be significantly less successful (by 30 to 60%) if we could not correct this condition. Massive PR is a reversal in most areas of life. Mini-PR is a block which kicks in during treatment and prevents the treatment from being complete. Recurring PR is a reversal, which returns as soon as it is corrected. Each of these variations of PR require their own special treatment. Of especial significance in TFT standard diagnostic procedures is that if a therapist is in PR, that therapist is unable to reveal the PR of a client. This problem, interestingly, does not appear in the Voice Technology™ method of diagnosis.

PSYCHOLOGICAL TRAUMA A psychological trauma is an experience or event that engenders significant emotional upset. The upset seems reasonably based and therefore is unlike other psychological problems. Examples of trauma are rape; robbery; friend murdered; mugging; loss of a loved one through death, or perhaps even worse, through rejection; loss of a cherished job; kidnapping of a child, witnessing traumatic events, etc. The appropriateness of the disturbing emotion accompanying the event appears to be a hallmark of the notion of trauma. One might not expect trauma to be so responsive to therapy as it is to TFT. This surprising fact carries important theoretical significance (see Chapter 1). Someone who loses his pen and is obsessed and very upset over this event (has nightmares, etc.), is not considered to have had a trauma, though it is an obvious psychological problem. In other words, it is not the upset per se that is relevant, but the appropriateness of the emotion to the event that is relevant.

QUANTUM LEAPS IN THERAPY It was apparent from the outset with TFT that not only is the therapy rapid and effective, but the manner of progress is unique, i.e., the progress takes place in large definite leaps with the client evidently not passing through intermediate stages of the problem. My first case, Mary, for example, moved from a 10 to a 1 instantly and did not pass through intermediate stages of intensity of the problem. One would expect that curing a life-long problem would not only be slow but might pass through a number of intermediate stages on the way to getting well. The typical case that begins with a SUD of 10 progresses with each stage of therapy to a 7, then a 4 and then a 1. The intermediate stages of intensity are typically bypassed.

REPRESSION A habit of avoidance of awareness of a painful emotion to the extent that the choice to be aware is lost. The repressed person usually remains unaware of the extent of emotional pain present unless the pain is overwhelming. Repressed people are as easily diagnosed and treated as anyone else except they do not know how they are doing (e.g., you don't know if the phobia is gone until they are *in* the phobic situation). The majority of people are not repressed and are aware of emotional pain when they attune the relevant thought field.

RESONANCE (see Tuning) The process that brings about attunement. A kind of physical bond that is brought about by a non-physical connection and may be operative in memory and tuning into a thought field. Proposed by Ninian Marshall (1960), the concept provides the foundation for Rupert Sheldrake's important notion of morphic resonance. Resonance is commonplace in the use of tuning forks and oscillating circuits used in radio and television; the oscillating circuitry in the receiver is adjusted to that of the transmission, and when they resonate, the program enters the receiver. When a person attunes a perturbed thought field, he or she become disturbed.

REVOLUTIONARY EXPERIMENT An experiment in science that reveals new facts which cannot be explained or accounted for by conventional or accepted notions current at the time of the experiment. For example, the clinical psychologist Martin Seligman, director of clinical training at the University of Pennsylvania, in his recent book *What You Can Change and What You Can't Change* states, "There are no quick fixes" and "Optimism is necessary for change to take place." (p. 253) Our reproducible experiments overturn both these cherished common-sense notions, as well as many others.

SCIENCE The proper function of science is to respect facts and to revise theories in the light of new facts. Science is by nature conservative and therefore slow in carrying out its proper function. It is typically quite difficult for conservative scientists to be able to *observe* easily demonstrable new facts (see apex problem).

SUD SUD stands for *subjective units of distress*, a scale introduced by Wolpe to quantify the degree of stress, pain, or disturbing emotion experienced by the client. In TFT the SUD is considered the bottom line by which therapy is evaluated for success. SUD may be an 11- or 10-point scale: 0 to 10 or 1 to 10. Behavioral indices of how people are responding to therapy may be quite misleading since many people can do things when pushed, but if their suffering remains intense, we do not consider this successful therapy. Many people in conventional therapies learn that they can withstand a great deal more suffering than they thought they could. Successful therapy, such as TFT, removes all traces of suffering.

THERAPY Therapy—or rather effective therapy—results in dramatic improvement in the way the client feels. The improvement referred to here is not merely behavioral change, which is relatively easy to obtain, but the removal of all traces of a psychological problem. We believe that effective therapy is a result of the subsumption (this appears to be the most appropriate term in this context), removal, collapse, elimination, or reduction of P's in a thought field, resulting in the elimination or reduction of negative emotions whether relevant to reality (considered appropriate and normal) or not (so-called and misnamed "neurotic"). As we learn in TFT, the root of the problem is not in the nerves but in the energy system of the body. The difference, after treatment, must be *clinically,* and not merely statistically, significant in order to qualify as successful therapy (see Adler, 1993). TFT is typically saltatory in its progression (saltus is a leap) or discontinuous in movement. This fact has led us to investigate quantum theory since the jumps are quantum-like. We currently believe that the actual treatment may occur at a quantum level. Presently it seems likely that a molecular bond is either broken or connected by the treatment or by natural maturation or healing.

THOUGHT FIELD (TF) The concept of thought field is a distinguishing characteristic of TFT. Other professions such as acupuncture, acupressure, chiropractic, medicine, dentistry, etc, involve work on the rather static body or being of the person. The dynamic and limitless potentiality of the thought field is what makes TFT a *psychological* treatment. When one is trained to diagnose TF's, it becomes immediately apparent that the structure of the TF creates dynamism in the individual. For example, it makes no difference to a dentist what you are thinking about when working on your teeth. For the TFT clinical psychologist, it makes all the difference in the world what is attuned. When the relevant TF is attuned it brings to the fore the specific P's and related information which are active in a problem and vital to understanding what is called for in the treatment situation. In order to diagnose and treat effectively, the appropriate TF must be attuned. Not attuning to the relevant TF is equivalent to asking a tailor to alter your trousers without bringing the trousers. A thought field is an imaginary scaffold upon which one may project or imagine causal entities such as perturbations. Empirical tests and clinical experience reveal the relevance and power of such imaginings, i.e., we then discover whether our imaginings are "on" or "off-line" with reality. There is overwhelming evidence for the on-line nature of our theoretical speculations. All human invention and discovery are initially in the human imagination and must be reality-tested to determine ultimate status. The ghosts of inventors of the airplane and the helicopter reside, in a sense, in these inventions. These inventions, to be deeply understood, are not just a combination of mechanical objects, not just dead machines. Only a fragmented manner of viewing results in this view.

Young children and animals do not have the ability to volitionally attune a thought field and for such cases the term *perceptual field* is more appropriate.

TRACKING Tracking refers to the procedure of observing the duration of a completely successful TFT treatment to see if any part of the problem returns. It is very important that a client call the TFT-trained therapist immediately should a problem, which has been completely eradicated, return. We find that this rare occasion is generally due to an ingestion of, or exposure to, an exogenous substance. A therapist trained in TFT diagnostic procedures can usually readily determine the substance. Diagnosis identifies and thus allows avoidance. After the substance is absent for a period of two months, giving the treated system a chance to heal, a repeat treatment will usually hold and then, after that time, the offending substance may no longer regenerate the psychological problem, though it is possible it may have other implications.

TRANQUILIZERS A means of *temporarily* blocking or reducing awareness of anxiety without addressing the cause of the problem. Tranquilizers appear to help by temporarily masking or hiding anxiety from awareness. It is my thesis that all addiction is addiction to some form of tranquilizer, whether chemical or behavioral.

TUNING (see Resonance) The process of bringing a particular thought associated with a problem into awareness. For example, a trauma victim will be asked to think about the trauma. Often trauma victims, clients with obsessive-compulsive disorder, addicts, and anxiety clients have INTRUSIVE TF's that enter under their own power and require no attunement. There can be no diagnosis or therapy without appropriate tuning. Animals or infants who have no choice in tuning must be *in* a situation that generates the appropriate tf, or rather perceptual field, in order to be diagnosed and treated effectively.

VOICE TECHNOLOGY™ The proprietary technology that allows for the rapid and precise diagnosis of P's by telephone through an objective and unique voice-analysis technology. The relevant (P) information can be demonstrated to be contained in holographic form within the voice. This fact allows diagnosis to be done with only a fraction of a second of the voice available. Language, choice of words, inflection and content are totally irrelevant to this astonishing process. The encoded information held in the voice is then decoded with precision and the empirical effectiveness of the discoveries so obtained is quite easy to demonstrate. This is not stress analysis, since stress is too vague to be useful in this context and can be assumed when a client requires help; it is rather a rapid decoding process of the relevant P information in the attuned thought field and contained within the voice.

WITHDRAWAL The acute anxiety experienced by an addict when deprived of his favored tranquilizer. Withdrawal is viewed in TFT as anxiety, unmasked. Even heroin addicts may be totally relieved of all physiologic (and, of course, psychological) symptoms with the TFT treatment for addictive urge or withdrawal. A chain-smoking cigarette smoker may be entirely unaware of the anxiety, which powers the need for cigarettes because the perpetually smoked cigarette *continually masks the anxiety.* The chain smoker never gives himself a chance to experience withdrawal. However, when deprived of a cigarette, the smoker becomes acutely aware of the underlying anxiety. One may therefore gauge the degree of an anxiety problem by the number of cigarettes smoked per day. The same reasoning applies to all addictions. The TFT algorithm for addiction withdrawal has a very high success rate, by which we mean the treatment eliminates the desire to consume a substance or engage in a behavioral addiction about 90% of the time. The TFT treatment is very effective in helping individuals addicted to prescribed tranquilizers,

· but this should always be done under the supervision of a knowledgeable professional.

APPENDIX B
Rap Song

I Just Can't Thought About It Anymore

Thought Field Therapy Rap
Mark Steinberg, Ph.D, VT—Therapist

Thought Field, Thought Field Therapy rap,
You gonna feel better when you know how to tap
The most effective cure on the whole darn planet
Once you've run through the entire gamut.

Think about it, think about it, get yourself zapped,
Negative emotions in a thought field trap.
Liberate yourself with some selective taps,
This is the Thought Field Therapy rap!

Therapy, therapy, I've had my fill.
They promise the world, but I tell 'em to chill.
Cause my problems weren't susceptible to kill
Until I used the Thought Field Therapy drill.

"I want to be over this problem," I declare.
I tap a little here, and I tap a little there.
I roll my eyes and I hum a little tune.
Amazingly, I feel much better pretty soon!

Thought Field Therapy makes very little sense
The apex problem makes its doubters real dense.
Though undeniably the problem before
I just can't thought about it anymore!

Perturbations, perturbations, gimme a break.
My energy field is beginning to ache.
My problem is irrational, but I can't shake
Reactions that continue for their own sake.

Talk about it, talk about it, does no good,
Guilty that I oughta, and knowing that I should.
Feeling pretty hopeless, but if only I could
Make myself feel better, I surely would.

Healing people tell me there's a measure of pain
In order to improve I gotta sustain.
With mostly discomfort and very little gain,
I tell the healing people their system is insane.

The method upon which Thought Field Therapy draws
Eradicates the problem's fundamental cause.
Removing perturbations and reversing flaws
According to natural energy laws.

Voice technology, ultimate psychology,
Diagnose the problem through energy topology
Cause of the disturbance is carried through your voice,
Now we can fix it without toxins, your choice.

Think about it, thought about it, feel upset.
With most interventions, such is what you get.
With Thought Field Therapy's quantum core
I just can't thought about the problem any more!

REFERENCES

Adler, T. (1993) Studies look at ways to keep fear at bay: Science Directorate report. *American Psychological Association, Monitor,* 24(11): 17.

Agar, W.E., Drummond, F.H., and Tiegs, O.W. (1942) Second report on a test of McDougall's Lamarckian experiment on the training of rats. *Journal of Experimental Biology* 19: 158-167.

American Psychiatric Association (1980) *Psychiatric Glossary.* Fifth Edition. Boston: Little Brown.

Arnold, M. (1960) *Emotion and Personality.* New York: Columbia University Press.

Aspect, A.; Dalibard, J.; and Roger, G. (1982) Experimental test of Bell inequalities using time-varying analyzers. *Physical Review Letters* 49: 1804.

Basset, C., Pawluk, R. Pila, A. (1974) Acceleration of Fracture Repair by Electromagnetic Fields. A Surgically Noninvasive Method. *NY Academy of Science,* 242-261.

Baeyer, Hans C. von. (1998) *Maxwell's Demon.* NY: Random House.

Beck, Aaron. (1976) *Cognitive Therapy and Emotional Disorders.* NY: International Universities Press, Inc.

Becker, Robert O. and Selden, G. (1987) *The Body Electric: Electromagnetism and the foundation of life.* NY: Morrow.

Bell, J.S. (1965) On the Einstein Podolsky Rosen Paradox. *Physics* 1:195-200.

Bishop, J.E. (1996) *The Wall Street Journal,* Monday, January 29, p. A9A.

Blaich, R. (1988) Applied Kinesiology and Human Performance. *Selected papers of the International College of Applied Kinesiology,* 1-15, Winter.

Blatner, D. (1997) *The Joy of Pi.* NY: Walker.

Bohm, D. (1957) *Causality and Chance in Modern Physics.* London: Routledge & Kegan Paul Ltd.

————. (1965; reissue 1989) *The Special Theory of Relativity.* NY: Addison-Wesley, Advanced Book Classics.

————. (1990) A new theory of the relationship of mind and matter. *Philosophical Psychology,* Vol. 3, No. 2, pp. 271-286.

Bohm, D. and Hiley, B.J. (1993) *The Undivided Universe: An ontological interpretation of quantum theory.* NY: Routledge.

Bosner, M.S. and Kleiger, R.E. (1995) Heart rate variability and risk stratification after myocardial infarction. In Malik, M. and Camm, A.J. (Eds) *Heart Rate Variability.* Armonk, NY: Futura.

Bouton, M. and Swartzentruber, D. (1991) Source of relapse after extinction in Pavlovian and instrumental learning. *Clinical Psychology Review,* 11:123-140.

Burr, H. S., and Northrop, F.S.C. (1935) The electro-dynamic theory of life. *Quarterly Review of Biology,* 10, 322.

Burr, H. S. (1947) Field theory in biology. *The Scientific Monthly,* 64: 217-225.

————. (1972) *Blueprint for Immortality: The electric patterns of life.* London: Neville Spearman.

Callahan, R. (1955) *The Measurement of Anxiety in a Group of Sixth Grade Children.* Doctoral dissertation, Syracuse University. Univ. Microfilms, Ann Arbor, MI.

Callahan, R. and Keller, J. (1957) Digit Span and Anxiety: an experimental group revisited. *American Journal of Mental Def.* 61: 581-582.

Callahan, R. (1960) Value orientation and psychotherapy. *Amer. Psychologist,* 15: 269-270 (cited by Albert Ellis [1962] in *Reason and Emotion in Psychotherapy.* NY: Lyle Stuart).

————. (1962) Validity of the CAP. *Perceptual and Motor Skills,* 14: 166.

————. (1978) *Test Manual for CAP (Callahan Anxiety Pictures): A projective test for experimental and clinical evaluation of anxiety in children.* Sunset Distributors, LA.

————. (1981a) A Rapid Treatment for Phobias, *Collected Papers, International College of Applied Kinesiology (ICAK).*

————. (1981b) Psychological Reversal. *Collected Papers of International College of Applied Kinesiology,* Winter, 79-96.

————. (1981c) The Amazing Love Pain Treatment (Trauma of loss). *Collected Papers, ICAK.*

Callahan, R. and Levine, K. (1982) *It Can Happen To You: The practical guide to romantic love.* NY: A & W.

Callahan, R. (1985) *Five Minute Phobia Cure.* Wilmington: Enterprise.

_____. (1987) Successful Treatment of Phobias and Anxiety by Telephone and Radio. *Collected Papers, ICAK,* Winter.

Callahan, R. with Perry, P. (1991) *Why Do I Eat When I'm Not Hungry?* New York: Doubleday.

_____. (1992) Paperback edition *Why Do I Eat When I'm Not Hungry?* New York: Avon.

Callahan, R. (1993a) *The Five Minute Phobia Cure: The Video.* La Quinta, CA.

_____. (1993b) *Love Pain: The Video.* La Quinta, CA.

_____. (1995a) A TFT Algorithm for the Treatment of Trauma. *Electronic Journal of Traumatology* 1(1).

_____. (1995b) The Apex Problem. Unpublished paper.

_____. (1995c) A TFT treatment for trauma. *Electronic Journal of Traumatology.*

_____. (1996) The Case of Mary: The first TFT case. *Electronic Journal of Traumatology,* 3(1).

_____. (1997) *TFT and Heart Rate Variability: An Interview With Fuller Royal, MD.* The Video. LaQuinta, Callahan Techniques.

Callahan, R. and Callahan, J. (1996) *TFT and Trauma.* LaQuinta, CA

Callahan Techniques® (1998) *Causal Diagnosis Home Study Course.* LaQuinta, CA.

Campbell, A. (1994) Cartesian Dualism and the concept of medical placebos, *Journal of Consciousness Studies,* 1(2): 230-233.

Carney, R.M., et al, (1995) Association of depression with reduced heart rate variability in coronary artery disease, *American Journal of Cardiology,* 76: 562-564.

Casolo, G. (1995) Heart rate variability in patients with heart failure. In Malik, M. and Camm, A.J. (Eds) *Heart Rate Variability.* Armonk, NY: Futura.

Chaplin, J.P. (1985) *Dictionary of Psychology.* NY: Dell, p. 342.

Chari, R. (1998) CT-TFT in a medical setting. *The Thought Field,* vol. 4, no. 2, pp. 1-2.

Cowen, R. (1999) Astronomers find planetary system. *Science News* (April 17), p. 244.

Crew, F.A.E. (1936) A repetition of McDougall's Lamarckian experiment. *Journal of Genetics,* 33: 61-101.

Daniel, S. (1997) Child treats child with TFT. *TFT Newsletter,* vol. 3, no. 2.

————. (1998) Ongoing Clinical Research with Callahan Techniques Thought Field Therapy Voice Technology™. *Thought Field Newsletter,* October.

Davies, Paul. (1988) *The Cosmic Blueprint.* NY: Touchstone.

Davies, P.C.W., and Julian Brown. (1989) *Superstrings: A Theory of Everything?* NY: Cambridge.

Einstein, A; Podolsky, B.; and Rosen, N. (1935) Can the quantum mechanical description of reality be considered complete? *Physical Review* 47:777-80.

Fallen, E.L. and Kamath, M.V. (1995) Circadian rhythms of heart rate variability. In Malik, M. and Camm, A.J. (Eds) *Heart Rate Variability*. Armonk, NY: Futura.

Feynman, Richard. (1967) *The Character of Physical Law*. Cambridge, MIT Press.

Figley, C. R. and Carbonell, J. L. (1994) The "Active Ingredient" Project: A systematic clinical demonstration study. Toward a clinically informed methodology for investigating clinical significance. Presented at the Active Ingredient Symposium, Tallahassee Memorial Regional Medical Center's Psychiatric Center, Tallahassee, September 9.

————. (1995) Treating PTSD: What approaches work best? Invited symposium at the Family Therapy Networker Conference, Washington, DC, March.

Foster, D. (1975) *The Intelligent Universe*. NY: Putnam.

————. (1985) *The Philosophical Scientists*. New York: Barnes and Noble.

Friedman, B.H., Thayer, J.F. (1998a) Anxiety and autonomic flexibility: a cardiovascular approach, *Biological Psychology*, 47(3): 243-63.

————. (1998b) Autonomic balance revisited: panic anxiety and heart rate variability. *Journal of Psychosomatic Res.*, 44(1): 133-51.

Freinkel, Andrew. (1994) Witness to the execution. *Science News*, September 24, 146(13): 200w.

Fry, E.S. (1993) *McGraw-Hill Encyclopedia of Physics* (2nd ed.). NY: McGraw-Hill

Gazzaniga, Michael. (1985) *The Social Brain.* NY: Basic Books.

_____. (1992) *Nature's Mind.* NY: Basic Books.

_____. (1998) *The Mind's Past,* Berkeley: University of California Press.

Gibson, E. and Walk, R. (1960). The visual cliff. *Scientific American,* April.

Gibson, J.G. (1962) *Psychological Review* 69: 477.

Goodwin, B. (1988) Science and philosophy of science. *Network—The Science and Medical Network Review.* No. 68 (December), pp. 44-45.

Goswami, Amit. (1993) *The Self-Aware Universe.* NY: Putnam.

Graham, Ian. (1999) Report on International Conference, Oslo, May, 1999—Treatment of Kosovan Refugees. *The Thought Field,* vol. 5, no. 1.

Graham, B., Rosenblum, S. and Callahan, R. (1958). Placebo Controlled Study of Reserpine in Maladjusted Retarded Children. *American Medical Association Journal of Diseases of Children,* 96: 690-695.

Grinberg-Zyleberbaum, J. (1988) *Creation of Experience. Mexico:* Instituto Nacional para el Estudio de la Conciencia.

Grinberg-Zyleberbaum, J. and Ramos, J. (1987) Patterns of interhemispheric correlation during human communication. *International Journal of Neuroscience,* 36: 41-54.

Grinberg-Zyleberbaum, J.; Delaflor, M.; Attie, L.; and Goswami, A. (1992) The EPR Paradox in the Human Brain. To be published.

Gross, Richard and Gubatosi-Klug, Rose A. (1996) Dec, *Journal of Biological Chemistry,* Washington University, School of Medicine, (also reported in *Science News,* Jan. 11, 1997, 151(2): 31)

Hameroff, S. R. (1974). Chi: A neural hologram? *American Journal of Chinese Medicine,* 2 (2) 163-70.

Ho, Mae-Wan. (1996) The biology of free will. *Journal of Consciousness Studies,* 3(3): 231-244.

Hon, E.H., and Lee, S.T. (1965) Electronic evaluations of the fetal heart rate patterns preceding fetal death: further observations. *American Journal of Obstetrics and Gynecology,* 87: 814-826.

Horne, Michael. (1991) in Lerner, R., and Trigg, G.L. *Encyclopedia of Physics.* NY: VCH.

Hugdahl and Kiarker. [(1981) Biological vs. experiential factors in phobic conditioning. *Behaviour Research and Therapy,* 15: 345-353.

Jacques, Jean. (1993) *The Molecule and its Double.* NY: McGraw Hill.

Joslin, G. (2000) Lab reports on immune system problem. *The Thought Field,* vol. 5, no. 2.

Jung, C.G. (1953) *The Archetypes and the Collective Unconscious.* London: Routledge and Kegan Paul.

Jammer, M. (1961) *Concepts of Mass—in Classical and Modern Physics.* Cambridge: Harvard University Press.

Kautzner, J. (1995) Reproducibility of heart rate variability measurement. In Malik, M. and Camm, A.J. (Eds) *Heart Rate Variability.* Armonk, NY: Futura.

Kawachi, I. et al. (1995) Decreased heart rate variability in men with phobic anxiety: data from the Normative Aging Study). *American Journal of Cardiology,* 75(14): 882-885.

Kienle, G.S. and Kiene, H. (1996) Placebo effect and placebo concept: a critical methodological and conceptual analysis of reports on the magnitude of the placebo effect. *Alternative Therapies in Health and Medicine,* 2(6): 39-53.

Koestler, Arthur. (1967) *The Ghost in the Machine.* NY: Viking-Penguin.

Komatusu T., Kimura T. Sanchala V., et al. (1992) Effects of fentanyl-diazepam-pancuronium anesthesia on heart rate variability: a spectral analysis. *Journal of Cardiothoracic Vascular Anesthesia,* 6: 444-448.

Langewitz, W. and Ruddel H. (1989) Spectral analysis of heart rate variability under mental stress. *Journal of Hypertension.*

Lashley, K.S. (1950) In search of the engram. *Symposia of the Society for Experimental Biology,* 4: 454-482.

LeDoux, J.E., L.M. Romanski, and A. E, Xagoraris. (1989) Indelibility of subcortical emotional memories. *Journal of Cognitive Neuroscience,* 1: 238-243.

LeDoux, J.E. (1994) Emotion, Memory and the Brain: The neural routes underlying the formation of memories about primitive emotional experiences, such as fear, have been traced. *Scientific American*, June, 50-57.

————. (1995) In search of an emotional system in the brain: Leaping from fear to emotion and consciousness. 1049-1061. In Gazzaniga, M. *The Cognitive Neurosciences*. Cambridge, MA, pp. 1049-1061.

Lehofer, M., et al. (1997) Major depression and cardiac autonomic control, *Biology of Psychiatry*, 42(10): 914-9.

Libchaber, Albert. (1996) Creative scientist. *Scientific American*, 199: 36-42.

Loewenstein, Werner R. (1999) *The Touchstone of Life: Molecular information, cell communication, and the foundations of life.* NY: Oxford University Press.

Malthus, T. (1798) *An Essay on the Principle of Population.* London: Johnson.

Malfatto, M. et al. (1996) In Malik, M. and Camm, A.J. (Eds) *Heart Rate Variability.* Armonk, NY: Futura.

Malik, M. and Camm, A.J. (1995) (Eds) *Heart Rate Variability.* Armonk, NY: Futura.

Malik, M. (Ed) (1997) *Clinical Guide to Cardiac Autonomic Tests.* Boston: Kluwer.

Mathias, C. and Alam, M. (1995) Circadian changes of the cardiovascular system and the autonomic nervous system: Observations in autonomic disorders. In Malik, M. and Camm, A.J. (Eds) *Heart Rate Variability.* Armonk, NY: Futura.

McDougall, W. (1927) An experiment for the testing of the hypothesis of Lamarck. *British Journal of Psychology*, 17: 267-304.

Marshall, Ian. (1989) Consciousness and Bose-Einstein condensates. *New Ideas in Psychology*, 7.

Marshall, Ninian. (1960) ESP and memory: A physical theory. *British Journal for the Philosophy of Science*, 10(40): 265-286.

Milius, Susan. (1999) The Search for Animal Inventors. *Science News*, June 5, vol. 155, no. 23, pp. 364-366.

Miller, M. (1996) Diet and Psychological Health. *Alternative Therapies*, 2(5): 40-48.

Miller, N.E. (1951) Learnable drives and rewards. in Stevens, S.S. (editor), *Handbook of Experimental Psychology*, NY: Wiley, 435-472.

_____. (1995) Clinical-Experimental Interactions in the Development of Neuroscience. *American Psychologist*, 50(11).

Milner, R. (1990) *The Encyclopedia of Evolution*. NY: Facts on File.

Milton, R. (1996) *Alternative Science: Challenging the myths of the scientific establishment*. Rochester, VT: Park Street Press.

Mindell, E. and Hopkins, V.H. (1998) *Prescription Alternatives*. New Canaan, CT: Keats.

Mindell, E. (1999) *Earl Mindell's Vitamin Bible for the 21*[st] *Century*. NY: Warner.

Moustakas, C. and Callahan, R. (1954) Reflections on Reflection of Feeling. *Journal of Family Living.*

Nahin, Paul J. (1998) *An Imaginary Tale: The story of $\sqrt{-1}$ (square root of minus 1).* Princeton NJ: Princeton University Press.

Nair, Gantum. (1996) *The Wall Street Journal,* Jan 16.

Newton, Roger. (1970) Particles that travel faster than light? *Science,* 167(3925): 1569-74a.

Nordenstrom, Bjorn. (1983) *Biologically Closed Electric Circuits: Clinical, experimental, and theoretical evidence for an additional circulatory system.* Stockholm: Nordic.

Peat, F. David. (1987) *Synchronicity.* NY: Bantam.

Peat, D. (1990) *Einstein's Moon: Bell's Theorem and the Curious Quest for Quantum Reality.* Chicago: Contemporary Books.

Penfield, W. (1975) *The Mystery of the Mind.* Princeton: Princeton University Press.

Pearsall, Paul. (1998) *The Heart's Code.* NY: Thorsons.

Penrose, R. (1990) *The Emperor's New Mind.* London: Oxford.

———. (1994) *Shadows of the Mind: A search for the missing science of consciousness.* NY: Oxford.

Plotkin and Odling-Smee. (1982) *Learning, Development and Culture: Essays in Evolutionary Epistemology.* NY: Wiley.

Popp, F.A., Warnke, U., Konig, H.L., and Peschka, W., Eds. (1989) *Electromagnetic Bioinformation.* Baltimore: Urban & Schwarzenberg.

Popper, Karl. (1997) Heroic Science. In Bolles, Edmund B. *Galileo's Commandment.* Freeman, NY.

Pribram, K.H. (1971) *Languages of the Brain.* Englewood Cliffs, NJ: Prentice-Hall.

Profet, Margie. (1991) The function of allergy: Immunological defense against toxins. *Quarterly Review of Biology,* 66, no. 1, March, pp. 23-62.

Rapp, Doris. (1991) *Is This Your Child?* NY: William Morrow.

Rosen, R. (1991) *Life Itself: A comprehensive inquiry into the nature, origin and fabrication of life.* NY: Columbia University Press.

Royal, Fuller. (1997) Video Interview on TFT and Heart Rate Variability, LaQuinta. CA: Callahan Techniques Ltd.

Rutter, V. (1994) Oops! A very embarrassing story. *Psychology Today,* March/April.

Sayers, B. (1973) Analysis of heart rate variability. *Ergonomics.* 16: 17-32.

Schmidt, G. and Morfill, G. (1995) Nonlinear methods for heart rate variability assessment. In Malik, M. and Camm, A.J. (Eds) *Heart Rate Variability.* Armonk, NY: Futura.

Schroedinger, Erwin. (1958, 1967) *What is Life?* NY: Cambridge.

Science News, Jan. 1997, 151, no. 2, p. 31 (see Gross, above).

Searle, John R. (1997) *The Mystery of Consciousness.* NY: New York Review of Books.

Seligman, M.E.P. (1971) Phobias and preparedness, *Behavior Therapy,* 2: 307-320

Seligman, M. (1994) *What You Can Change and What You Can't.* NY: Knopf.

Shannon, Claude E. (1948) A mathematical theory of information. *Bell System Technology Journal,* 27: 279-423; 623-656.

———. (1949) Communication in the presence of noise. Proc. *J.R.E.* 37: 10.

———. (1956) Zero-error capacity of noisy channels. *I.R.E.* Trans. I.T. 2:8.

Sheldrake, R. (1987) *A New Science of Life.* Los Angeles: Tarcher (originally published in 1981).

———. (1989) *The Presence of the Past.* NY: Vintage.

———. (1990) The Habits of Nature—III (Memory). Lecture given at Big Sur, Dolphin Tapes, CA.

———. (1994) *Seven Experiments That Could Change the World: A Do-It-Yourself Guide to Revolutionary Science.* London: Fourth Estate.

Singer, D. and Ori, Z. (1995) Changes in heart rate variability associated with sudden cardiac death. In Malik, M and Camm, A.J. (Eds) *Heart Rate Variability.* Armonk, NY: Futura.

Smith, C.W. (1999) Personal communication.

Sokal, Alan and Bricmont, Jean. (1998) *Fashionable Non-sense: Postmodern Intellectuals' Abuse of Science.* Picador, NY.

Stapp, Henry P. (1977) *Nuovo Cimento* 40B, 191.

_____. (1993) *Mind, Matter, and Quantum Mechanics.* NY: Springer-Verlag.

Stewart, Ian (1998) *Life's Other Secret.* NY: Penguin.

Sylvia, Claire (1997) *A Change of Heart.* NY: Warner.

Task Force of the European Society of Cardiology and the North American Society of Pacing and Electrophysiology. (1996) (Chairman, Marek Malik, Ph.D., MD) *Circulation,* 93:1043-1065.

Travis, C., McLean, B., and Ribar, C. (1989) *Environmental Toxins: Psychological, Behavioral, and Sociocultural Aspects.* 1973-1989 Washington, DC: American Psychological Association.

Vanoli, E., Adamson, P., Cerati, D., and Hull, S. (1995) Heart rate variability and risk stratification post-myocardial infarction: physiological correlates. In Malik, M. and Camm, A.J. (Eds) *Heart Rate Variability.* Armonk, NY: Futura.

Varela, F.J. (1996) Neurophenomenology: A Methodological Remedy for the Hard Problem. *Journal of Consciousness Studies,* 3(4): 330-349.

Wade, J. (1990) The Effects of the Callahan Phobia Treatment Technique on Self Concept. *Doctoral disserta-*

tion, The Professional School of Professional Psychology, San Diego.

Walther, D. (1988) *Applied Kinesiology: Synopsis.* Pueblo, CO: Systems DC.

Wigner, E. (1961) The probability of the existence of a self-reproducing unit. In Polyani, M. (Ed) *The Logic of Personal Knowledge.* London: Routledge and Paul.

Williams, G.C. and Nesse, R.M. (1991) The dawn of Darwinian medicine. *Quarterly Review of Biology,* 66, No. 1, 1-22.

Wylie, M.S. (1996) Going for the Cure. *Family Therapy Networker,* July/Aug.

Wolpe, J. and Wolpe, D. (1988) *Life Without Fear: Anxiety and its Cure.* Oakland: New Harbinger.

Yap, Y. and Camm, A. (1998) Clinical perspective. In Malik, M. (Ed) *Clinical Guide to Cardiac Autonomic Tests.* Kluwer, Netherlands.

Yeragani, V.K. et al. (1991) Heart rate variability in patients with major depression, *Psychiatry Res* 37(1): 35-46.

_____. (1998) Decreased heart-period variability in patients with panic disorder: a study of Holter ECG records, *Psychiatry Res* 78(1-2): 89-99.

Yin, Jerry. (1995) Molecules of Memory, *Science News* April 22, vol. 147, no. 16, pp. 241-256.

Young, A.M. (1976) *The Geometry of Meaning.* Lake Oswego, OR: Robert Briggs.

_____. (1979a). *The Reflexive Universe.* Lake Oswego, OR: Robert Briggs.

_____. (1979b) *The Bell Notes* Lake Oswego, OR: Robert Briggs.

_____. (1980) *Which Way Out* Lake Oswego, OR: Robert Briggs.

_____. (1990) *Mathematics, Physics, and Reality.* Lake Oswego, OR: Robert Briggs.

Youngson, R.M. (1994) *The Guinness Encyclopedia of Science.* Middlesex, England: Guinness.

INDEX

A

Alcohol, electric effect 84, 85
Algorithms 16, 17, 43, 47, 49, 52, 65, 109, 164, 179, 188, 191, 234, 280
Amouraphobia 34
Anorexia 188
Anticipatory anxiety 161, 162, 273
Apex problem 95, 96, 98, 99, 100, 101, 102, 103, 104, 105, 106, 107, 108, 109, 110, 116, 124, 133, 176, 193, 196, 273, 274, 296
Applied Kinesiology 75, 78, 175, 225, 255, 256, 258
Architecture of treatment 192
Aspect, Alain 214, 215
Atavism 126, 151, 274

B

Becker, Robert O. 76, 83
Bell, John 213, 214
Blaich, Robert 77, 78, 285
Bohm, David 45, 54, 55, 63, 137, 169, 179, 213, 282
Burr, Harold Saxton 71

C

Cancer 10, 11, 79, 80, 81, 82, 83, 101, 127, 129, 132, 200
Canfield, Jack viii
Causal Diagnosis 16, 26, 28, 31, 45, 46, 47, 48, 49, 53, 65, 75, 117, 120, 145, 154, 157, 165, 166, 167, 173, 183, 190, 192, 201, 202, 239, 242, 250, 253, 258, 260, 265, 266, 269, 271, 282
Causality 55, 63, 64, 274
Chari, Roopa 90
Child abuse 38

Q

R

S

**Now you can help yourself achieve optimal
mental health with the Callahan Techniques®,
Thought Field Therapy self-help programs.**

For the last half of the twentieth century Dr. Roger Callahan has researched and developed simple and effective self-help procedures to assist you with the challenges and stresses of daily life. Based on this continual research and development he has created many simple algorithms for your use. Most of Dr. Callahan's products are not available in stores so for more information about these products or the revolutionary new findings in Heart Rate Variability call, write, fax, or visit our web sites:

Dr. Roger J. Callahan
Callahan Techniques, Ltd.
Thought Field Therapy Training Center
78-816 Via Carmel
La Quinta, CA 92253
1-800-359-CURE (2873)—phone
1-760-360-5258—fax
001 760-564-1008—phone for international inquiries
www.selfhelpuniv.com (self-help site)
www.tftrx.com (professional site)

Home Training:
Callahan Techniques® Thought Field Therapy—
Step A—Basic TFT Training—Self Study course

Presented by Dr. Roger J. Callahan, Founder of TFT, teaches the step-by-step process for determining precise protocols for whatever the presenting problems (the same methods by which all of the above algorithm packages were developed). Includes training manual, two training videos, one demonstrational video, six audio tapes and our new Hand-Held Flip Chart. Now Only $499.00. For more information about Step A and any of our other training programs contact us at the numbers given above.